easy yoga

any age • any place • any time

Jude Reignier

Consultant Osteopath
Sean Durkan

Illustrated by
Juliet Percival

CONNECTIONS
BOOK PUBLISHING

A CONNECTIONS EDITION

This edition published in Great Britain in 2007 by
Connections Book Publishing Limited
St Chad's House, 148 King's Cross Road
London WC1X 9DH
www.connections-publishing.com

British Library Cataloguing-in-Publication data available on request.

ISBN 978-1-85906-218-0

1   3   5   7   9   10   8   6   4   2

Phototypeset in Meta using QuarkXPress on Apple Macintosh
Printed in China

Contents

Introduction

I have been teaching yoga for 10 years, both in classes and on a one-to-one basis. My clients have been diverse, including children, expectant mothers and those with special needs. I have found that most of my clients have little time to practise yoga, so they require their routines to be short and simple but effective. This book is written with those people in mind, and for anyone who doesn't have 1½ to 2 hours a day to practise but is keen to experience the benefits that a good yoga routine can offer.

Yoga can be practised in almost any calm environment where you won't be disturbed. Make sure any televisions or computers are switched off and the lighting is soft. If the floor is uncarpeted, use a large towel or, if possible, a yoga mat, which you should be able to purchase from any good sports shop. Wear loose, comfortable clothing and keep your feet bare – this will make it much easier to grip the floor.

How to use this book
The book consists of one 45-minute session, followed by two sessions of 20 minutes and then two of 10 minutes. The postures in the full 45-minute sequence work the whole body system, massaging and stimulating the internal organs while gently stretching, firming and toning the muscles and ligaments. The shorter sessions will energize or relax you, depending on which one you choose. Each one is made up of twelve or six of the postures shown in the 45-minute sequence.

When you've become familiar with the instructions given in the book, you may wish to practise without stopping to consult the book mid-session. If so, the wall chart shown on the inside of the book jacket will provide a handy memory aid should you need it. Whichever sequence you choose, practise the postures in the order shown.

If possible, practise the 45-minute session twice a week. You will start to see benefits after just a few weeks. If you wish, however, you could incorporate this session into your daily routine, but do take one day off every week to give your body a rest. The 20- and 10-minute sessions can be practised every day, or even twice a day. You will see results quicker the more you practise. After completing any of the shorter routines, always relax for at least 5 minutes (20-minute session) or 2 minutes (10-minute session) by lying or sitting quietly with your eyes closed.

Never push your body beyond its natural limit. Take each posture only as far as your body allows. Once you have memorized the sequences, the postures will flow together without any thought. And, as you gain confidence, you will be able to let your body and mind go, and this way you will achieve maximum benefit.

Deep breathing

Normal, or passive, breathing involves movement of the diaphragm. When we breathe in, the diaphragm moves down, increasing the ribcage capacity and allowing the lungs to expand to take in more oxygen. As we breathe out, the diaphragm moves up, forcing out carbon dioxide.

An efficient breathing cycle results in a balance between the oxygen and carbon dioxide levels in the blood, which enhances the functions of the body. Shallow breathing often manifests itself as hyperventilation. This is usually a result of prolonged stress or poor posture, and means that we're breathing out too much carbon dioxide, altering the normal body chemistry and disturbing the body's acid–alkaline balance. It also affects the bloodflow to the heart and brain, producing symptoms such as pins and needles, dizziness, headaches, muscle spasms, depression, asthma and insomnia.

Yoga helps us to concentrate on our breathing and encourages us to breathe more deeply, thereby improving the efficiency of our vital functions.

Massaging the organs

As the diaphragm moves up and down, it compresses and stretches the internal organs. This enhances the circulation of the blood and lymphatic drainage, which is essential for good health. The instructions for each posture in this book include a diagram illustrating the internal organs that are being massaged (*see below*). This allows you to see at a glance whether the posture mainly benefits the organs above or below the diaphragm, and is a good reminder that yoga does much more than toning and stretching the muscles.

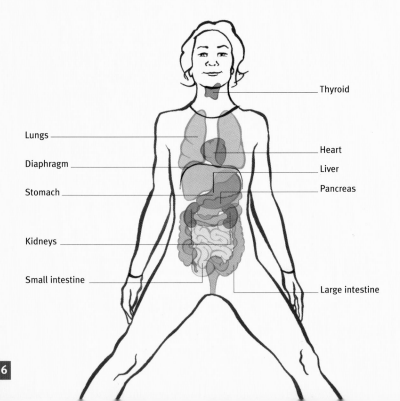

Thyroid

Lungs

Heart

Diaphragm

Liver

Stomach

Pancreas

Kidneys

Small intestine

Large intestine

Stretching the muscles

At the stage of each posture where the muscles become stretched, the illustrations show a dotted line to demonstrate which muscles are being worked (*see below*). This will not only tell you which parts of your body you are exercising, but will also act as a guide to whether you are performing the posture correctly as you should feel the muscles indicated become taut. If this isn't the case, relax, check that you're following the instructions correctly and assume the posture again. If you feel pain at any time, do not continue the posture.

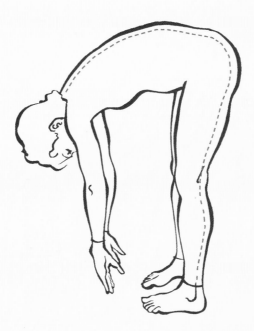

full-length sequence

45-MINUTE SESSION

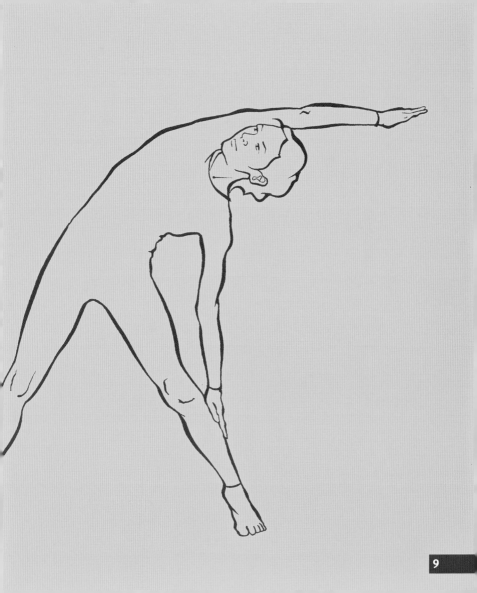

① Focus your breath

Improves circulation to all organs • Relaxes muscles and ligaments • Relieves stress

Lie down and gently close your eyes. Slowly inhale through the nose and focus on your breath as it travels down the throat and into the bottom of the lungs and ribcage. Be aware of your lungs and ribcage expanding and your spine lengthening. You will feel the abdomen rise.

Exhale through your nose. Feel the abdomen fall. The out-breath should be longer than the in-breath.

Surrender the weight of your body into the ground. Let go of your thoughts. Focus your breathing.

- **The exhalation holds the key to relaxation. The more stale air you exhale, the more fresh air you can inhale, the deeper your breathing, the quieter the mind.**

  Focus your breath ... relax ... relax.

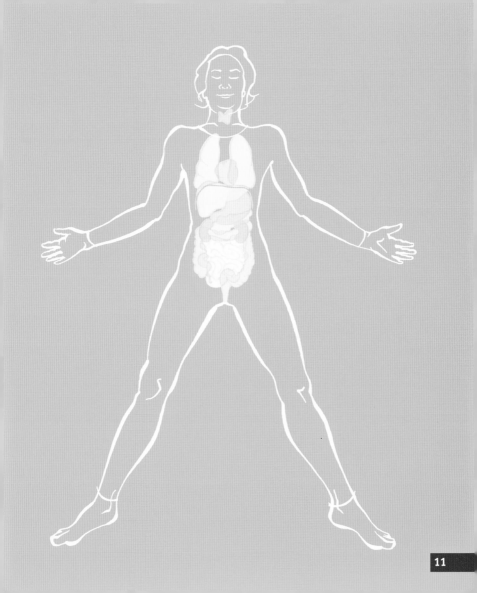

❷ The mountain

Improves circulation to all organs • Tones the arms • Firms the abdomen • Improves posture

1   Stand with your feet hip-width apart, heels turned out slightly. Stretch your arms out in front of you and link your fingers.

2   Inhale to prepare.

3   As you exhale, stretch your arms up above your head and root your feet firmly into the ground. Become aware of the opposite stretch creating space around your waist.

▶   Focus your breath as you stretch gently in the posture. Hold the stretch for 1 minute. Then release your arms and place them by your sides.

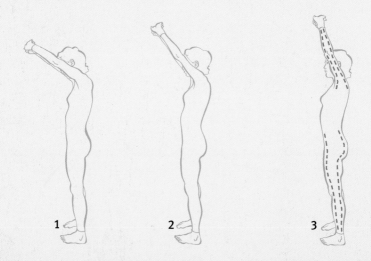

1   2   3

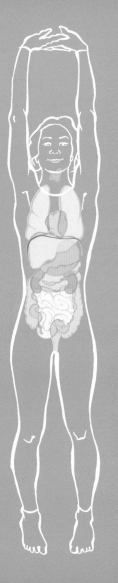

❸ Letting go

Stimulates the liver, kidneys and intestines • Helps to relieve stress, fatigue and indigestion • Stretches the calf muscles and hamstrings

Caution: Do not attempt this posture if you suffer from high blood pressure.

1   Standing with your feet hip-width apart and your heels turned out slightly, relax your body forwards, your arms hanging down.

2   Inhale as your body relaxes down.

3   As you exhale, drop your chin to your chest and slowly continue to release your spine, one vertebra at a time. Do not bounce. Root your feet firmly into the ground to keep your legs strong, and open the backs of the knees without locking them. Let go of the tension in the upper body.

▶   Exhale to release the spine, then the shoulders, arms, fingers, neck, face, jaw and eyes. Focus your breath as you hold the posture. Hold for 1 minute, then slowly come up to a standing position.

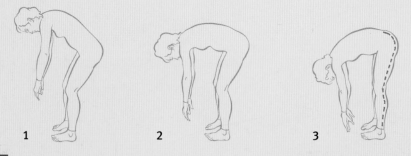

1   2   3

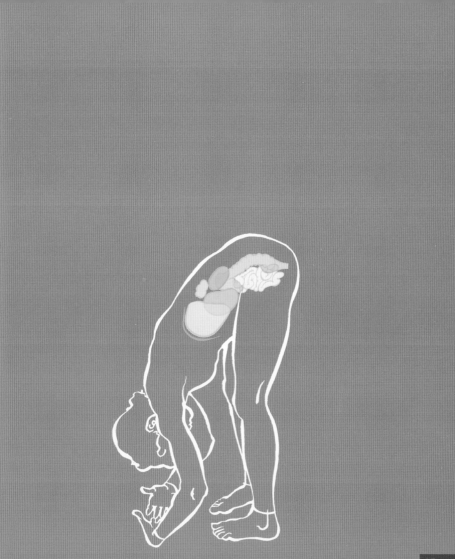

❹ The standing fish

Corrects rounded shoulders • Expands lungs • Tones the arms • Helps to relieve asthma, lethargy and anxiety

1 Standing with your feet hip-width apart, heels turned out slightly, link your fingers together behind your back.

2 Inhale to prepare.

3 As you exhale, slowly lift the centre of the chest and open the shoulders back, pulling the arms down. Root your feet firmly into the ground, keeping your legs strong and the backs of the knees open.

▶ As you focus your breath in the posture, your chest should be lifted and fully open and your arms pulled back. Hold for 1 minute. Then slowly release your arms and allow them to rest by your sides.

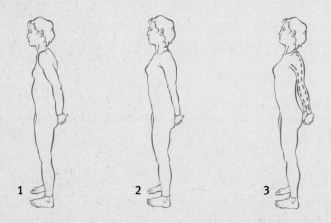

1   2   3

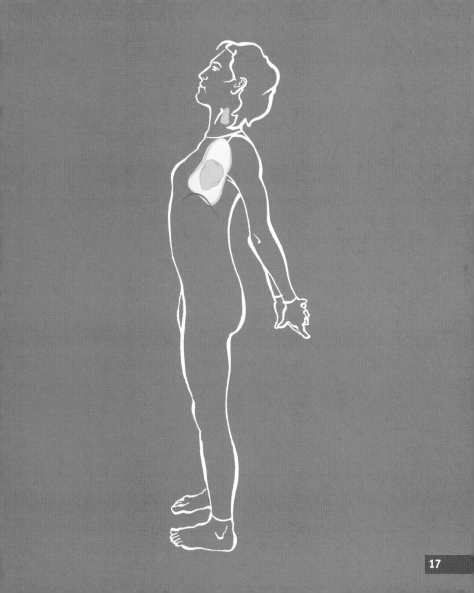

❺ The cobbler

Improves circulation to all organs • Stretches the inner thighs and groin • Opens the chest and shoulders • Helps to relieve asthma and menstrual discomfort

1 Lie on your back and bend your knees up towards the ceiling so that your feet are a few inches away from your buttocks, your feet and ankles together. Spread your arms to an angle of 45 degrees to your body. Keep your head centred and your chin tucked in. Inhale to prepare.

2 As you slowly exhale, begin to open your knees.

3 Continue to open your knees, keeping the lower back pressed into the ground.

▶ Focus your breath as you allow the hips to open fully. Hold for 1 minute. Then slowly bring the knees together.

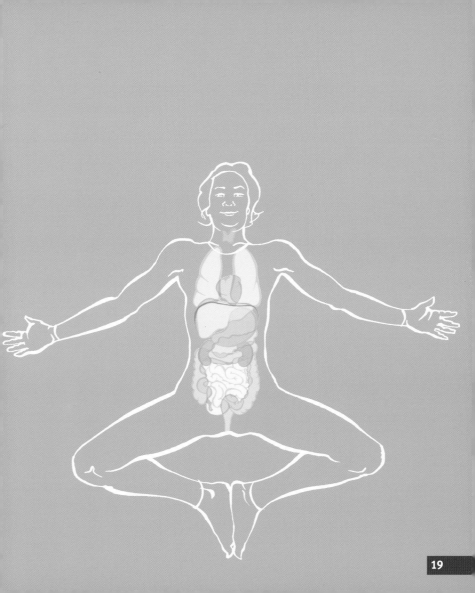

❻ The hip roll

Stimulates the liver, kidneys and intestines • Helps to relieve trapped nerves, indigestion and constipation • Stretches the thighs • Releases tension in the spine • Opens the shoulders and chest • Helps to relieve asthma

Caution: Do not attempt this posture if you are pregnant.

1 Lying on your back, feet together, bend your knees up to the ceiling. Bring your arms out, level with your shoulders, palms facing up. Your head should be centred and your chin tucked in. Inhale to prepare.

2 As you slowly exhale, drop your knees to the left as far as is comfortable. As you do so, turn your head to the right, twisting the spine.

3 Inhale. Then slowly exhale, bringing the knees and head back to centre.

▶ Repeat to the other side. Continue for 2 minutes, twisting to one side, then the other. To finish, bring the knees and head back to centre.

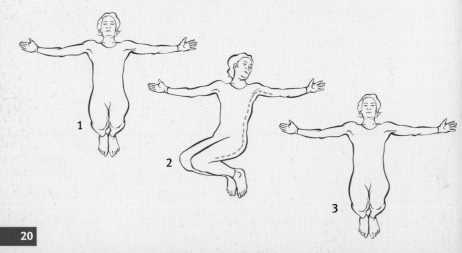

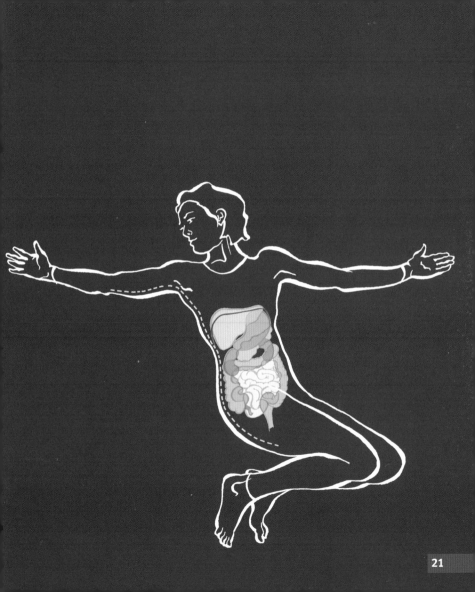

❼ The pelvic tilt

Stimulates the thyroid • Expands the lungs • Stretches the neck and thighs • Strengthens the lower back and abdominal muscles • Helps to relieve asthma, menstrual discomfort and back pain

Caution: Avoid this posture if you're pregnant or have a neck injury.

1 Lie on your back with your knees bent and your feet hip-width apart, heels turned out slightly. Place your arms by your sides, palms down. Keep your head centred and your chin tucked in. Inhale to prepare.

2 Slowly exhale, lifting your tail bone off the ground as you do so.

3 Lift each vertebra off the ground one by one until you reach the shoulder blades.

▶ Root your feet firmly into the ground. Become aware of your chest opening as you push the spine up as far as is comfortable. Inhale. Then exhale as you slowly lower the spine, one vertebra at a time – upper spine, central spine, lower spine, tail bone. Repeat the pelvic tilt for 1 minute.

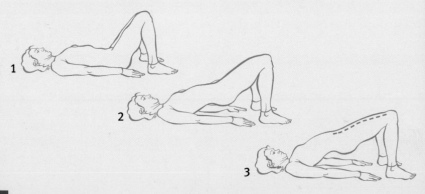

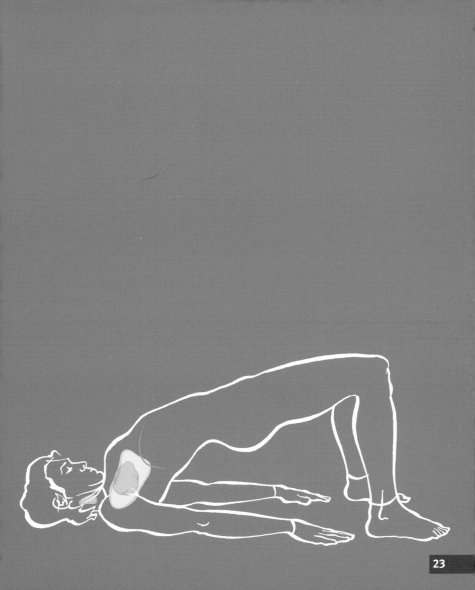

❽ The big toe

Improves circulation to all organs • Stretches the hamstrings and calf muscles • Tones the abdominal muscles • Improves flexibility in the hips • Helps to relieve back pain, indigestion and constipation

1 Lie on your back with your chin tucked into your neck, and your lower back pressed into the ground. Inhale to prepare.

2 Slowly exhale, raising your legs off the ground. Use your hands to support your upper legs.

3 Focusing your breath, raise the legs as far as you can manage, using your hands to guide them. Extend through the heels to open up the backs of the legs.

▶ Grab hold of your toes and gently pull your legs towards you as far as is comfortable, keeping the backs of the knees open. Hold the posture for 1 minute. Slowly lower your legs to the floor.

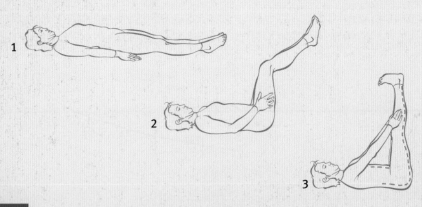

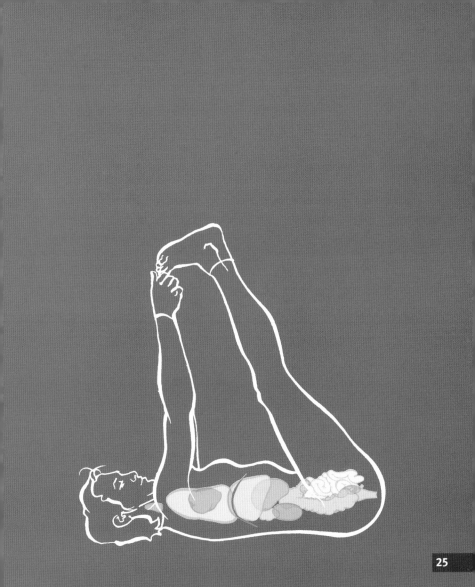

⑨ The half dog

Stimulates the liver, kidneys and intestines • Helps to relieve lower back pain and indigestion • Tones the arms • Opens the chest, central spine and shoulders • Helps to relieve asthma

1 On all fours, position your hands in line with the shoulders, and your knees hip-width apart. Inhale to prepare.

2 As you exhale, widen the arms and move them forwards on the floor.

3 Slowly drop the chest and shoulders towards the ground, ensuring that the hips remain in line with the knees.

▶ Focus your breath, allowing the chest and shoulders to open and the spine to lengthen. Hold the posture for 1 minute, or less if it becomes uncomfortable. Then return to the starting position.

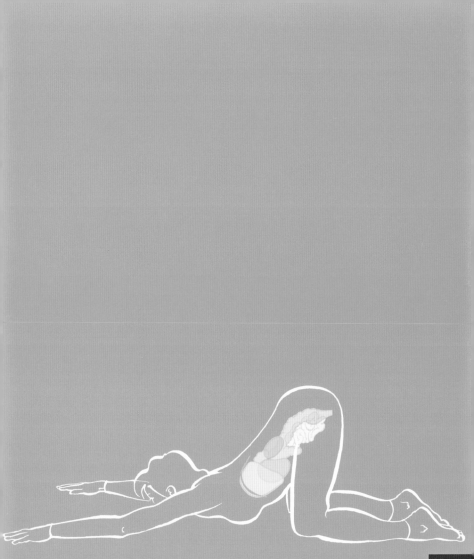

⑩ The cobra

*Improves circulation to all organs • Tones the arms and abdomen •
Expands the lungs • Helps to relieve asthma, menstrual discomfort,
constipation and indigestion*

Caution: Avoid this posture if you're pregnant or suffer from lower back pain.

1 Lie on your front with your forehead down, legs together and hands
   in line with the outside of your shoulders. Inhale to prepare.

2 As you exhale, slowly lift the forehead, chin and neck, pushing your
   hands into the ground.

3 Continue to push, lifting the chest and ribs. Draw the elbows down
   towards the waist, pull the shoulders back and down, and open the chest.

▶ Focus your breath. Hold the posture for 30 seconds. Then slowly lower
   the ribs, chest, neck, chin and finally the forehead, back to the floor.
   Then repeat.

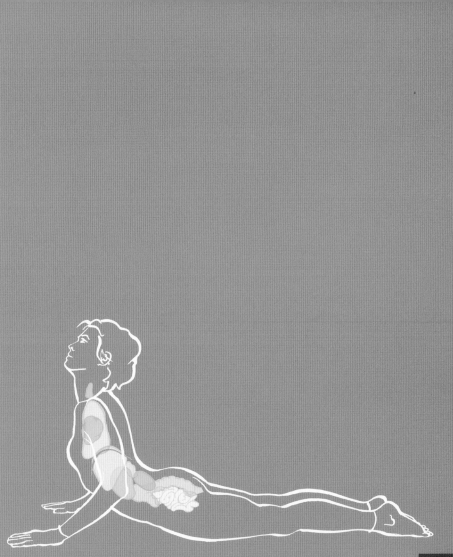

⑪ The locust

Stimulates the liver, kidneys and intestines • Helps to relieve indigestion • Stretches the thighs • Strengthens the lower back

Caution: Avoid this posture if you're pregnant or suffer from lower back pain.

1 Lie on your front with your throat lengthened along the floor. Place your arms by your sides, palms facing up, shoulders relaxed.

2 Inhale, slowly lifting your right leg off the ground. Ensure that your hips remain flat to the floor – do not allow them to twist. Exhale as you slowly lower your leg.

▶ Repeat with the left leg. Complete the locust 5 times with each leg.

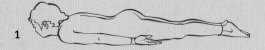

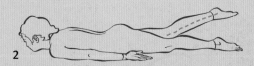

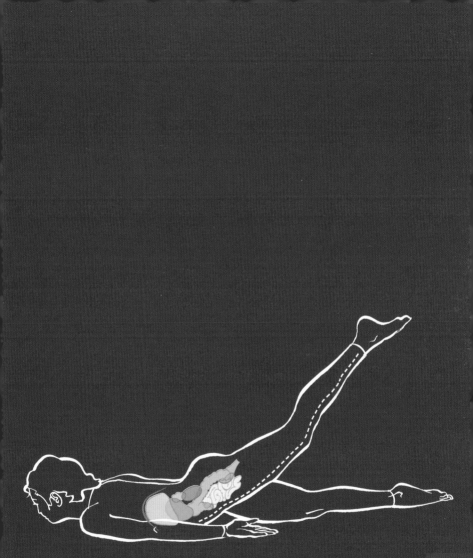

31

⑫ The dog

Improves circulation to all organs • Stretches the calf muscles, hamstrings, spine, arms and hands • Helps to relieve back pain, headache, fatigue and indigestion

Caution: Do not attempt this posture if you have high blood pressure.

1 On all fours, position your hands in line with the shoulders, knees hip-width apart. Inhale to prepare.

2 As you exhale, bring your weight onto the toes, and slowly lift the knees.

3 Push your tail bone up and out. With your heels turned outwards slightly, extend them to the floor to open out the backs of the knees.

▶ Lengthening the legs fully, relax the neck and face. Focus your breath. Hold the posture for 1 minute. Then slowly return to the starting position.

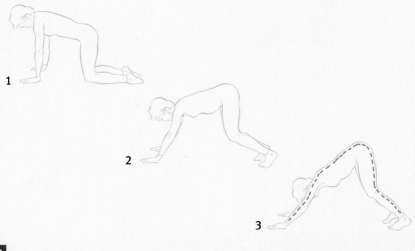

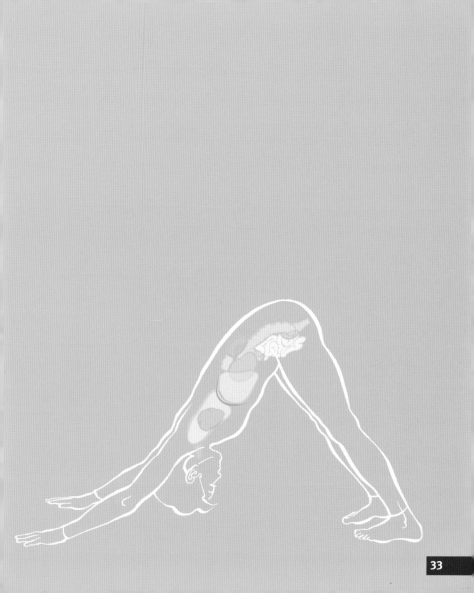

⑬ The wide-leg triangle

Stimulates the liver, kidneys and intestines • Helps to relieve indigestion • Improves balance and spinal flexibility • Tones the legs • Stretches the arms • Strengthens the lower back and abdominal muscles

1 Stand with your feet wide apart, toes pointing forwards. Raise your right arm so that it brushes against your ear, fingers pointing to the ceiling. Inhale to prepare.

2 With your face turned into the raised arm, slowly exhale. As you do so, stretch your arm and torso to the left, keeping the left arm straight, by your side.

3 As you stretch, root your right foot firmly into the ground. Ensure that your hips are pointing forwards – do not allow them to twist. If you experience any pain in your sides, stop.

▶ Focus your breath. Hold the posture for 30 seconds. Then slowly return to the standing position and release the arm. Repeat to the other side.

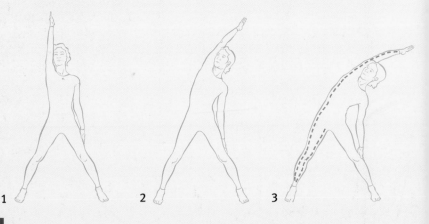

1   2   3

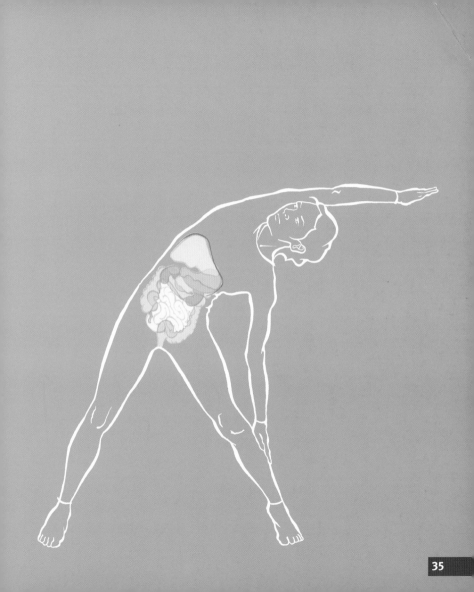

⑭ The triangle variation

Stimulates the kidneys, liver and intestines • Helps to relieve fatigue, stress, stiffness in the shoulders and indigestion • Stretches the calf muscles and hamstrings • Tones the arms

Caution: Do not attempt this posture if you suffer from high blood pressure or lower back pain.

1 Stand with your feet wide apart, toes pointing forwards. Root your feet firmly into the ground. Position your hands behind your back and link your fingers together. Inhale to prepare.

2 As you exhale, slowly bend forwards with the spine relaxed.

3 Continue to bend, taking your arms over your head.

▶ Focus your breath. Hold the posture for 1 minute. Then slowly return to the standing position and release the arms.

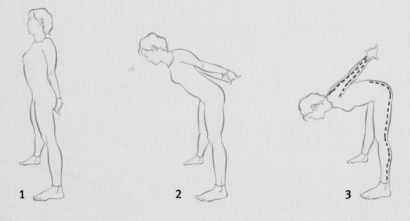

1   2   3

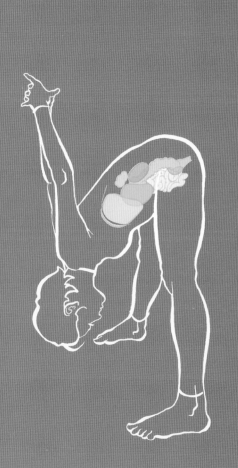

⑮ The warrior

Improves circulation to all organs • Stretches the groin and inner thighs • Strengthens the legs • Opens the chest • Helps to relieve asthma and stress • Improves stamina and balance

1 Stand with your feet as far apart as is comfortable. Slowly turn your left foot out 90 degrees, keeping your hips pointed forwards.

2 Raise both arms out to the sides level with your shoulders, keeping the shoulders relaxed. Your palms should be turned downwards. Inhale to prepare.

3 As you exhale, slowly bend the left knee, keeping your body centred.

▶ Continue to bend until your leg forms a right-angle. Turn your head to the left – you should be able to feel the lightness in your upper body and the strength in your legs. Focus your breath. Hold the posture for 30 seconds. Slowly return to the starting position, then repeat to the other side.

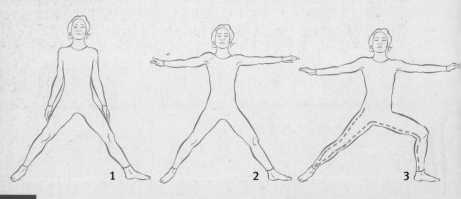

1   2   3

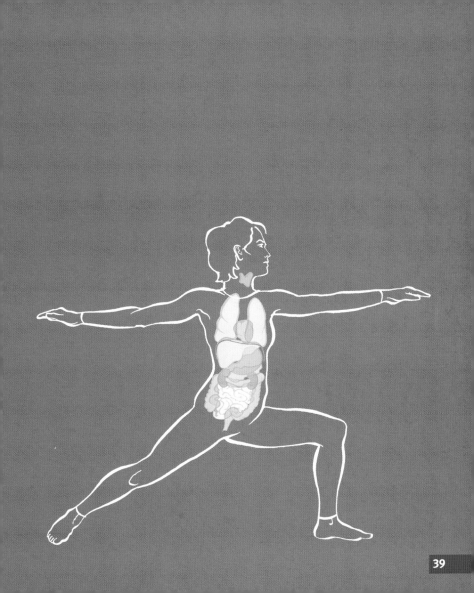

⑯ The stork

Improves circulation to all organs • Stretches the thighs and arms •
Expands the lungs • Opens the hips • Helps to relieve asthma and stress
• Improves concentration and balance

1 Stand with your feet hip-width apart, toes pointing forwards, arms by your sides.

2 Bend your right leg up behind you and take hold of the ankle with your right hand. Raise your left arm so that your fingers point towards the ceiling. Your arm should gently brush your ear. Inhale to prepare.

3 Root the left foot firmly into the ground and, as you exhale, slowly lean forwards and push your right foot up to the ceiling. Make sure your hips are straight throughout – do not allow them to twist. Keep the grounded leg strong and straight.

▶ Focus your breath. Hold the posture for 1 minute. Then slowly release the leg, and relax the arm. Repeat to the other side.

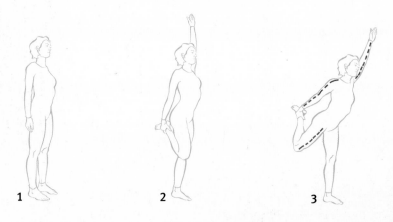

1   2   3

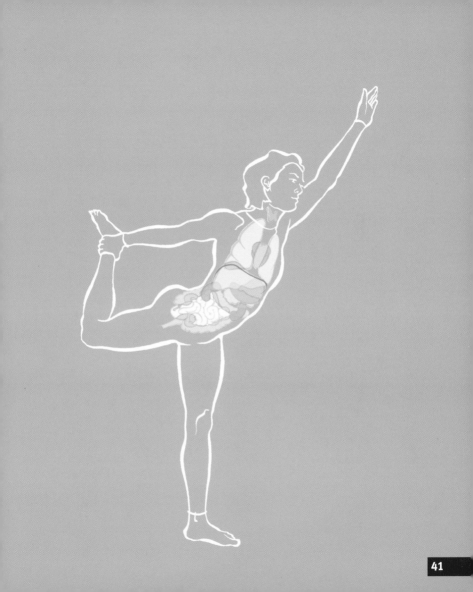

⓱ The shoulder stand

Improves circulation to all organs • Stretches the neck • Stimulates the thyroid • Invigorates the body • Tones the abdominal muscles • Helps to relieve asthma, indigestion and varicose veins

Caution: Avoid this posture if you're pregnant or suffering from high blood pressure, neck pain or injury, or pins and needles in the arms or hands.

1 Lie on your back with your legs together, arms by your sides, palms face down. Keep your head centred and your chin tucked in. Inhale to prepare.

2 As you exhale, slowly raise your legs until they're positioned over your torso. Then, pressing your hands into the floor, begin to lift your hips.

3 Support your back with both hands, fingers turned into the spine, thumbs around the hips. Continue to lift the legs and hips, gradually moving the hands up the back as the distance between your head and feet increases. Keep your elbows tucked in to distribute the weight evenly and avoid pressure on the neck and shoulders.

▶ Focus your breath. Hold the posture for 1–2 minutes, or less if it becomes uncomfortable. To release, slowly take your legs to an angle of 45 degrees over your head, and press your palms into the floor. Slowly lower the spine to the floor, one vertebra at a time, followed by the legs.

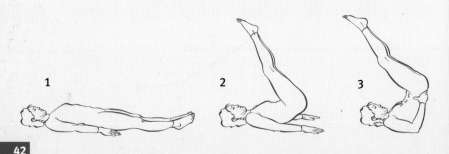

1   2   3

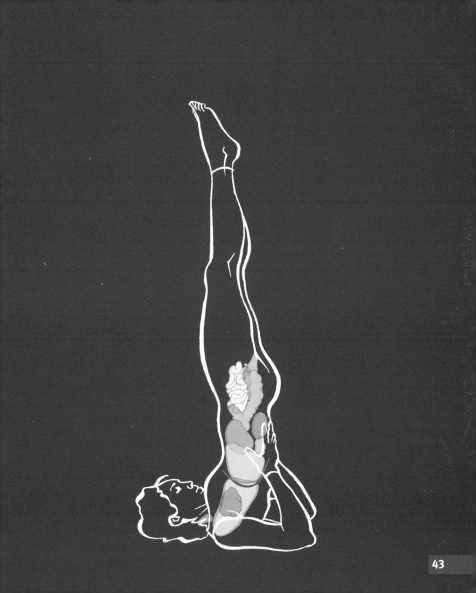

⑱ The plough

Improves circulation to all organs • Stretches the neck, spine, hamstrings and calf muscles • Stimulates the thyroid • Helps to relieve asthma, neck and back pain, indigestion and constipation

Caution: Avoid this posture if you're pregnant or suffering from high blood pressure, neck pain or injury, or pins and needles in the arms or hands.

1 Lie on your back with your legs together. Place your arms by your sides, palms down. Your head should be centred, chin tucked in. Inhale.

2 As you exhale, press your hands into the ground. Slowly raise your legs until they're positioned over your torso, then raise your hips.

3 Support your back with both hands, fingers turned into the spine and thumbs towards the hips. Tuck your elbows in. Slowly take your legs over your head. The aim is for your feet to touch the floor behind your head, but do not force them if it starts to feel uncomfortable.

▶ Tuck your toes in and straighten your legs. Keep the hips lifted and the chin tucked in to take the weight away from the neck and shoulders. Focus your breath. Hold the posture for 1 minute. To release, press your palms into the floor, then slowly lower the spine one vertebra at a time from the shoulders to the tail bone. Then gently lower the legs.

1

2

3

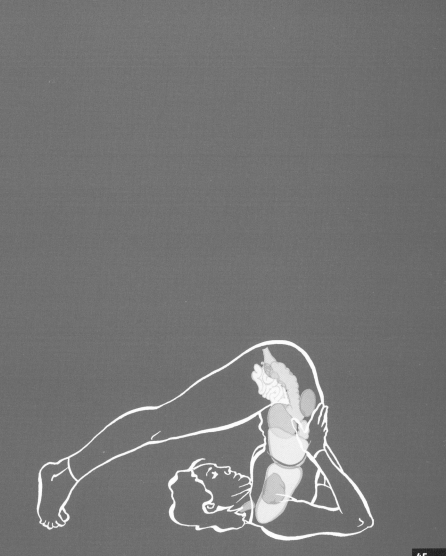

⑲ The fish

Expands the lungs • Stimulates the thyroid • Stretches the neck and spine •
Opens the shoulders • Tones the arms • Helps to relieve asthma and stress

**Caution: Avoid this posture if you have a neck injury or suffer from pins
and needles in the arms or hands.**

1 Lie on your back with your legs together. Place your arms by your
sides, palms down. Keep your head centred, chin tucked in.

2 With your arms straight, position your hands underneath your buttocks
so that your hands are side by side, pointing towards the thighs. Inhale
to prepare.

3 Exhale, pressing your elbows into the floor. As you do so, arch your
back and lift your chest.

▶ Slowly lower your head back until the top of the head touches the floor.
Focus your breath. Hold the posture for 1 minute. To release, gently lift
your head, then lower your body, returning your arms to your sides.

1

2

3

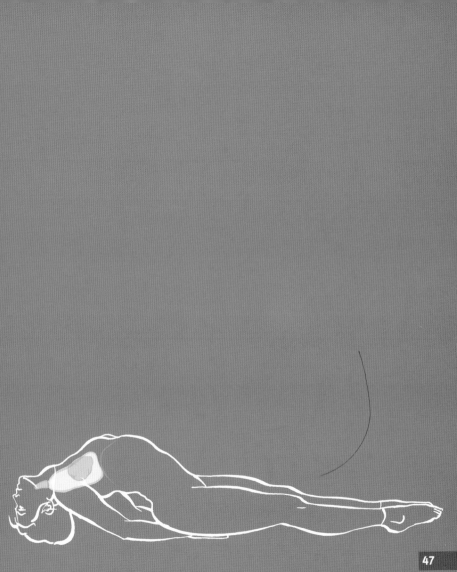

㉒ Tense and release

Improves circulation to all organs • Releases tension in the muscles

1 Lie on your back with your feet wide apart, arms at 45 degrees to the body. Your palms should be facing upwards, and your head centred. Tuck your chin in and gently close your eyes.

2 As you inhale, tense your hands and feet, making fists with your hands and curling your toes.

3 Lift your head, arms, hands, legs and feet 5–8 cm (2–3 in) off the floor. Feel the tension throughout your body. Hold for 10 seconds.

▶ As you exhale, let go completely. Release your head, arms, hands, legs and feet. Your whole body should feel totally relaxed. Focus your breath for 1 minute.

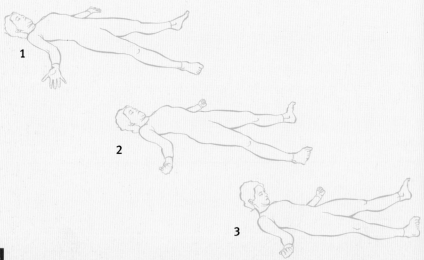

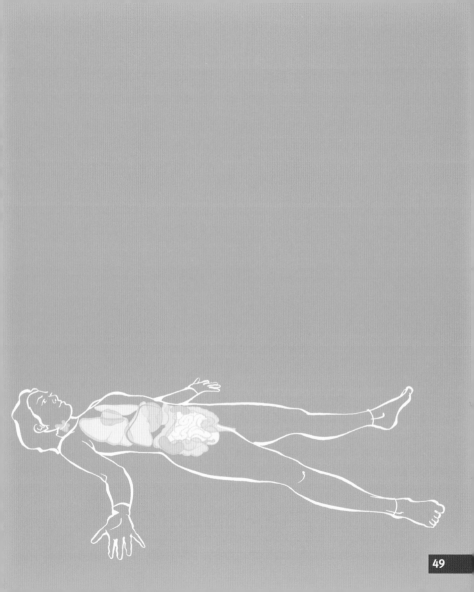

㉑ Auto-suggestion relaxation

Lowers the pulse rate • Reduces energy loss and stress build-up • Allows the whole body to rest • Relaxes the brain • Clears the mind

Lie on your back with your feet wide apart, arms at 45 degrees to your body, palms facing upwards. Keep your head centred and your chin tucked in. Focus your breath for a few minutes. As you do so, visualize your body with your mind's eye.

Taking your attention to the feet, silently say to yourself, 'I relax my feet … I relax my feet …. my feet are relaxed.'

Then take your attention to your legs and silently say to yourself, 'I relax my legs … I relax my legs … my legs are relaxed.'

One by one, repeat this process for the hips, spine, shoulders, arms, hands, fingers, neck, jaw, eyes, face, skull, liver, kidneys, stomach, intestines, pancreas, lungs, thyroid and heart.

When your heart is relaxed, let go … focus your breath. Your mind, body and spirit, your very being, should now feel totally relaxed.

Just lie still for 10 minutes. Focus on nothing but the calmness of your body and the quietness of your mind.

Inhale, and slowly bring your legs together and your arms above your head. Pressing the lower back into the floor, exhale, and stretch out the whole body as far as you can. Feel the stretch in your arms, legs, back and neck. Then slowly stand up.

■ **By concentrating the mind on specific parts of the body, we're able to fully relax those areas. This is the perfect way to end the sequence.**

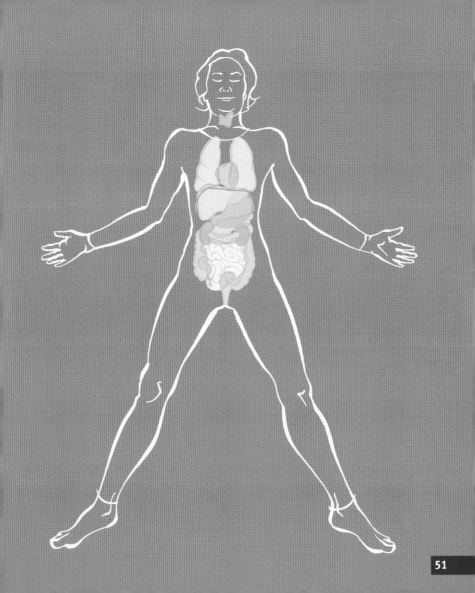

energize
and unwind

20-MINUTE SESSIONS

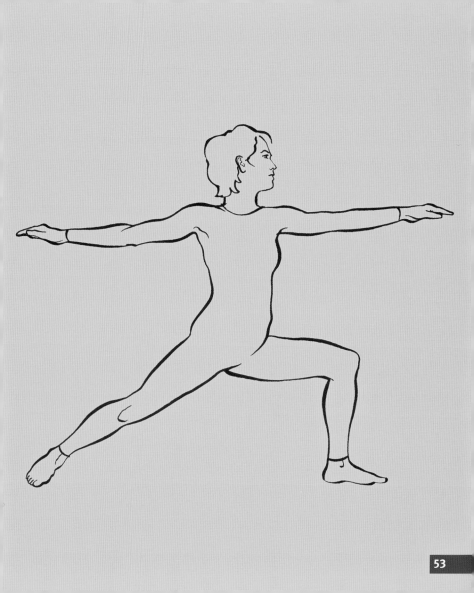

❶ The mountain

Improves circulation to all organs • Tones the arms • Firms the abdomen • Improves posture

1 Stand with your feet hip-width apart, heels turned out slightly. Stretch your arms out in front of you and link your fingers.

2 Inhale to prepare.

3 As you exhale, stretch your arms up above your head and root your feet firmly into the ground. Become aware of the opposite stretch creating space around your waist.

▶ Focus your breath as you stretch gently in the posture. Hold the stretch for 1 minute. Then release your arms and place them by your sides.

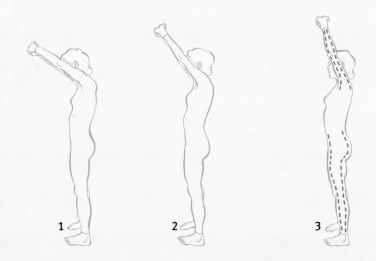

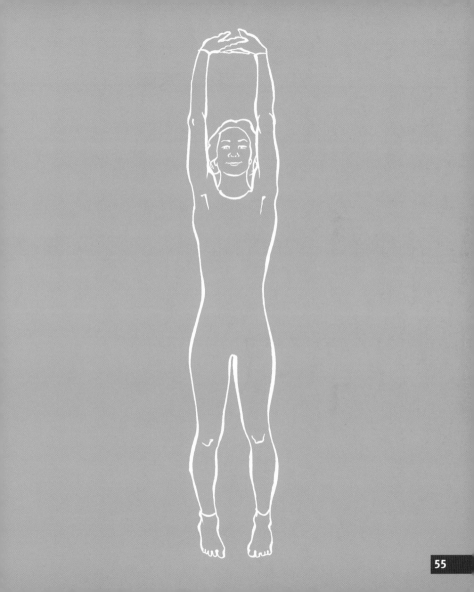

② Letting go

Stimulates the liver, kidneys and intestines • Helps to relieve stress, fatigue and indigestion • Stretches the calf muscles and hamstrings

Caution: Do not attempt this posture if you suffer from high blood pressure.

1 Standing with your feet hip-width apart and your heels turned out slightly, relax your body forwards, your arms hanging down.

2 Inhale as your body relaxes down.

3 As you exhale, drop your chin to your chest and slowly continue to release your spine, one vertebra at a time. Do not bounce. Root your feet firmly into the ground to keep your legs strong, and open the backs of the knees without locking them. Let go of the tension in the upper body.

▶ Exhale to release the spine, then the shoulders, arms, fingers, neck, face, jaw and eyes. Focus your breath as you hold the posture. Hold for 1 minute, then slowly come up to a standing position.

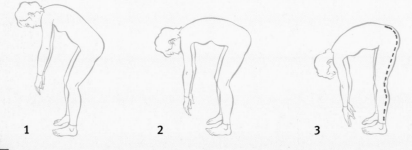

1   2   3

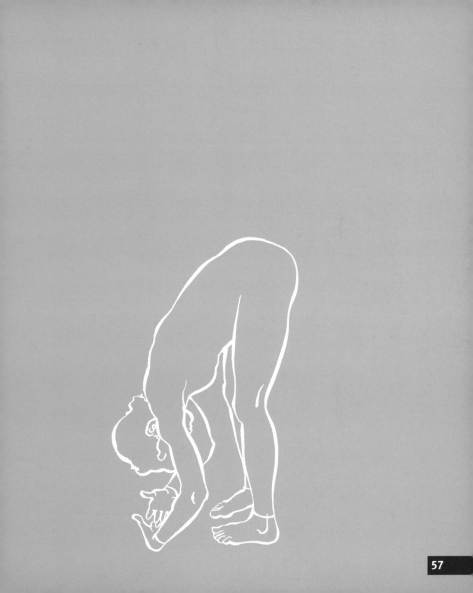

❸ The standing fish

Corrects rounded shoulders • Expands lungs • Tones the arms • Helps to relieve asthma, lethargy and anxiety

1 Standing with your feet hip-width apart, heels turned out slightly, link your fingers together behind your back.

2 Inhale to prepare.

3 As you exhale, slowly lift the centre of the chest and open the shoulders back, pulling the arms down. Root your feet firmly into the ground, keeping your legs strong and the backs of the knees open.

▶ As you focus your breath in the posture, your chest should be lifted and fully open and your arms pulled back. Hold for 1 minute. Then slowly release your arms and allow them to rest by your sides.

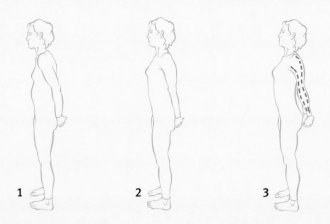

1   2   3

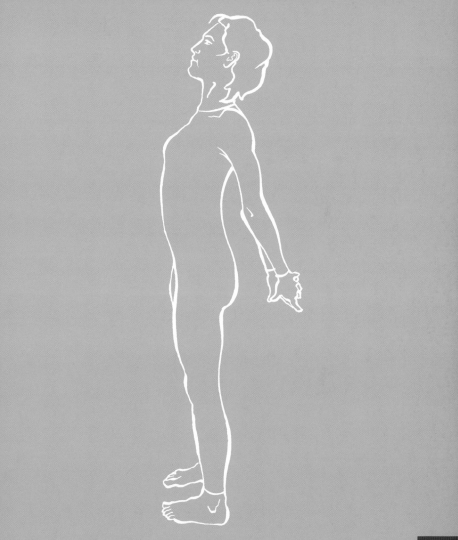

❹ The triangle variation

Stimulates the kidneys, liver and intestines • Helps to relieve fatigue, stress, stiffness in the shoulders and indigestion • Stretches the calf muscles and hamstrings • Tones the arms

Caution: Do not attempt this posture if you suffer from high blood pressure or lower back pain.

1 Stand with your feet wide apart, toes pointing forwards. Root your feet firmly into the ground. Position your hands behind your back and link your fingers together. Inhale to prepare.

2 As you exhale, slowly bend forwards with the spine relaxed.

3 Continue to bend, taking your arms over your head.

▶ Focus your breath. Hold the posture for 1 minute. Then slowly return to the standing position and release the arms.

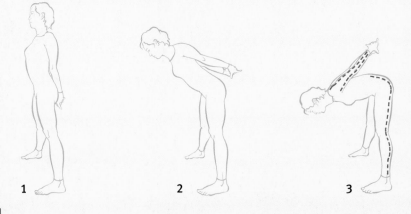

1   2   3

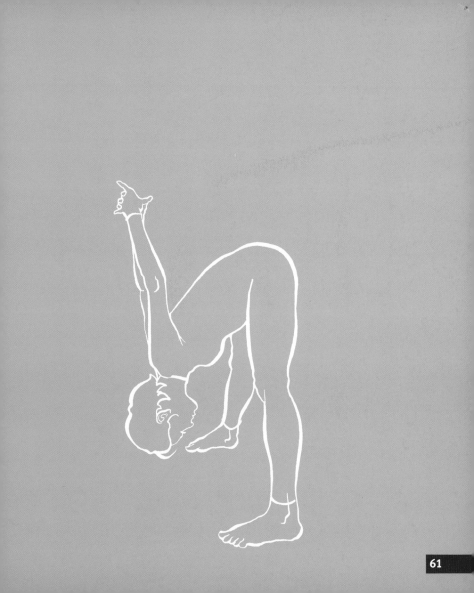

❺ The cobra

Improves circulation to all organs • Tones the arms and abdomen •
Expands the lungs • Helps to relieve asthma, menstrual discomfort,
constipation and indigestion

Caution: Avoid this posture if you're pregnant or suffer from lower back pain.

1 Lie on your front with your forehead down, legs together and hands
   in line with the outside of your shoulders. Inhale to prepare.

2 As you exhale, slowly lift the forehead, chin and neck, pushing your
   hands into the ground.

3 Continue to push, lifting the chest and ribs. Draw the elbows down
   towards the waist, pull the shoulders back and down, and open the chest.

▶ Focus your breath. Hold the posture for 30 seconds. Then slowly lower
   the ribs, chest, neck, chin and finally the forehead, back to the floor.
   Then repeat.

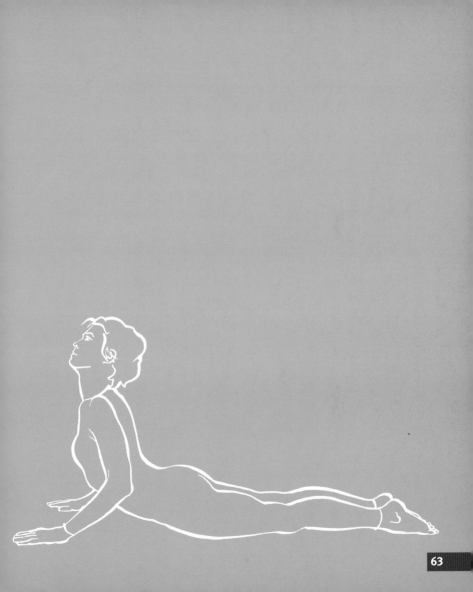

❻ The locust

Stimulates the liver, kidneys and intestines • Helps to relieve indigestion • Stretches the thighs • Strengthens the lower back

Caution: Avoid this posture if you're pregnant or suffer from lower back pain.

1 Lie on your front with your throat lengthened along the floor. Place your arms by your sides, palms facing up, shoulders relaxed.

2 Inhale, slowly lifting your right leg off the ground. Ensure that your hips remain flat to the floor – do not allow them to twist. Exhale as you slowly lower your leg.

▶ Repeat with the left leg. Complete the locust 5 times with each leg.

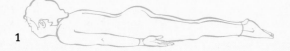

1

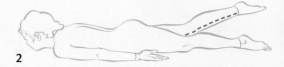

2

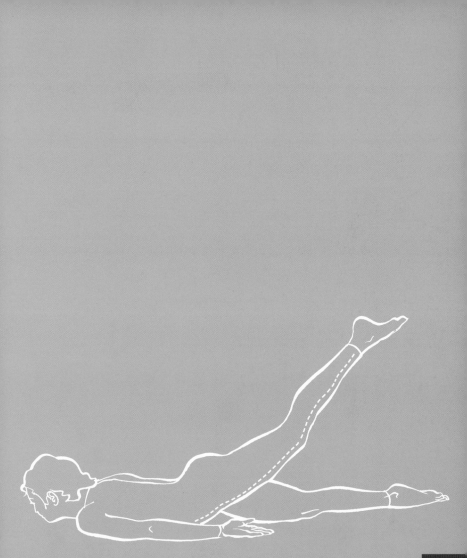

❼ The dog

Improves circulation to all organs • Stretches the calf muscles, hamstrings, spine, arms and hands • Helps to relieve back pain, headache, fatigue and indigestion

Caution: Do not attempt this posture if you have high blood pressure.

1 On all fours, position your hands in line with the shoulders, knees hip-width apart. Inhale to prepare.

2 As you exhale, bring your weight onto the toes, and slowly lift the knees.

3 Push your tail bone up and out. With your heels turned outwards slightly, extend them to the floor to open out the backs of the knees.

▶ Lengthening the legs fully, relax the neck and face. Focus your breath. Hold the posture for 1 minute. Then slowly return to the starting position.

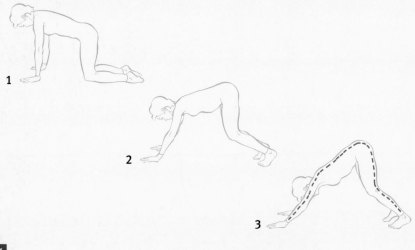

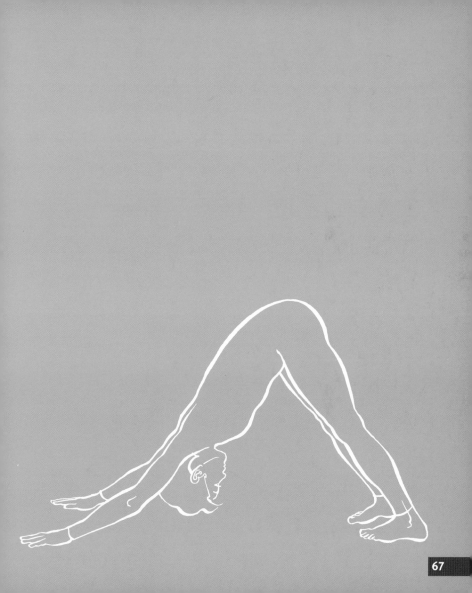

⑧ The wide-leg triangle

Stimulates the liver, kidneys and intestines • Helps to relieve indigestion • Improves balance and spinal flexibility • Tones the legs • Stretches the arms • Strengthens the lower back and abdominal muscles

1 Stand with your feet wide apart, toes pointing forwards. Raise your right arm so that it brushes against your ear, fingers pointing to the ceiling. Inhale to prepare.

2 With your face turned into the raised arm, slowly exhale. As you do so, stretch your arm and torso to the left, keeping the left arm straight, by your side.

3 As you stretch, root your right foot firmly into the ground. Ensure that your hips are pointing forwards – do not allow them to twist. If you experience any pain in your sides, stop.

▶ Focus your breath. Hold the posture for 30 seconds. Then slowly return to the standing position and release the arm. Repeat to the other side.

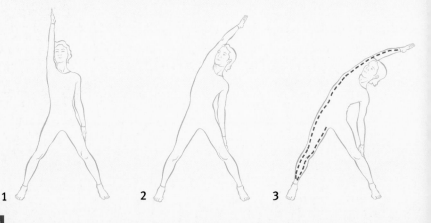

1   2   3

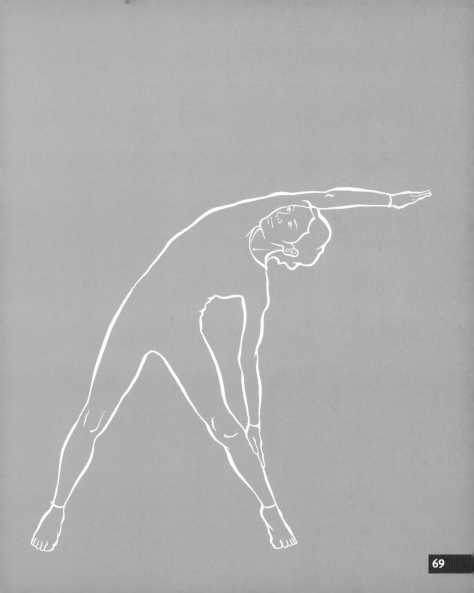

⑨ The warrior

Improves circulation to all organs • Stretches the groin and inner thighs • Strengthens the legs • Opens the chest • Helps to relieve asthma and stress • Improves stamina and balance

1   Stand with your feet as far apart as is comfortable. Slowly turn your left foot out 90 degrees, keeping your hips pointed forwards.

2   Raise both arms out to the sides level with your shoulders, keeping the shoulders relaxed. Your palms should be turned downwards. Inhale to prepare.

3   As you exhale, slowly bend the left knee, keeping your body centred.

▶   Continue to bend until your leg forms a right-angle. Turn your head to the left – you should be able to feel the lightness in your upper body and the strength in your legs. Focus your breath. Hold the posture for 30 seconds. Slowly return to the starting position, then repeat to the other side.

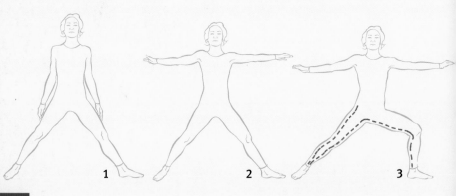

1   2   3

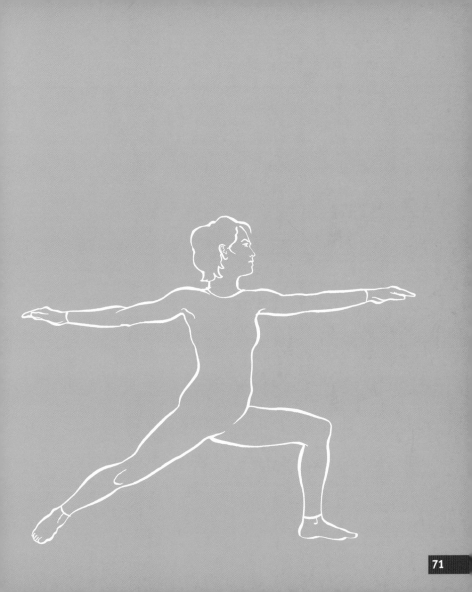

⑩ The big toe

Improves circulation to all organs • Stretches the hamstrings and calf muscles • Tones the abdominal muscles • Improves flexibility in the hips • Helps to relieve back pain, indigestion and constipation

1 Lie on your back with your chin tucked into your neck, and your lower back pressed into the ground. Inhale to prepare.

2 Slowly exhale, raising your legs off the ground. Use your hands to support your upper legs.

3 Focusing your breath, raise the legs as far as you can manage, using your hands to guide them. Extend through the heels to open up the backs of the legs.

▶ Grab hold of your toes and gently pull your legs towards you as far as is comfortable, keeping the backs of the knees open. Hold the posture for 1 minute. Slowly lower your legs to the floor.

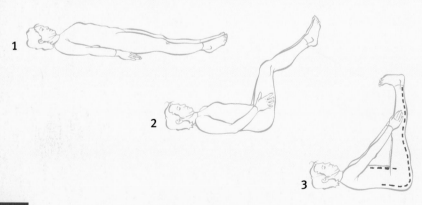

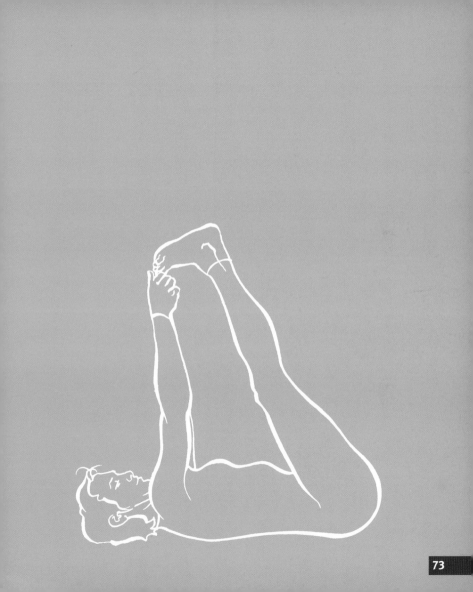

⑪ The shoulder stand

Improves circulation to all organs • Stretches the neck • Stimulates the thyroid • Invigorates the body • Tones the abdominal muscles • Helps to relieve asthma, indigestion and varicose veins

Caution: Avoid this posture if you're pregnant or suffering from high blood pressure, neck pain or injury, or pins and needles in the arms or hands.

1 Lie on your back with your legs together, arms by your sides, palms face down. Keep your head centred and your chin tucked in. Inhale to prepare.

2 As you exhale, slowly raise your legs until they're positioned over your torso. Then, pressing your hands into the floor, begin to lift your hips.

3 Support your back with both hands, fingers turned into the spine, thumbs around the hips. Continue to lift the legs and hips, gradually moving the hands up the back as the distance between your head and feet increases. Keep your elbows tucked in to distribute the weight evenly and avoid pressure on the neck and shoulders.

▶ Focus your breath. Hold the posture for 1–2 minutes, or less if it becomes uncomfortable. To release, slowly take your legs to an angle of 45 degrees over your head, and press your palms into the floor. Slowly lower the spine to the floor, one vertebra at a time, followed by the legs.

1   2   3

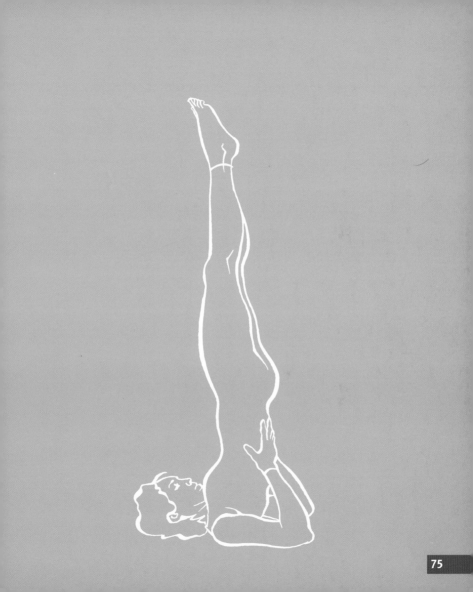

⑫ The fish

Expands the lungs • Stimulates the thyroid • Stretches the neck and spine • Opens the shoulders • Tones the arms • Helps to relieve asthma and stress

Caution: Avoid this posture if you have a neck injury or suffer from pins and needles in the arms or hands.

1 Lie on your back with your legs together. Place your arms by your sides, palms down. Keep your head centred, chin tucked in.

2 With your arms straight, position your hands underneath your buttocks so that your hands are side by side, pointing towards the thighs. Inhale to prepare.

3 Exhale, pressing your elbows into the floor. As you do so, arch your back and lift your chest.

▶ Slowly lower your head back until the top of the head touches the floor. Focus your breath. Hold the posture for 1 minute. To release, gently lift your head, then lower your body, returning your arms to your sides.

1

2

3

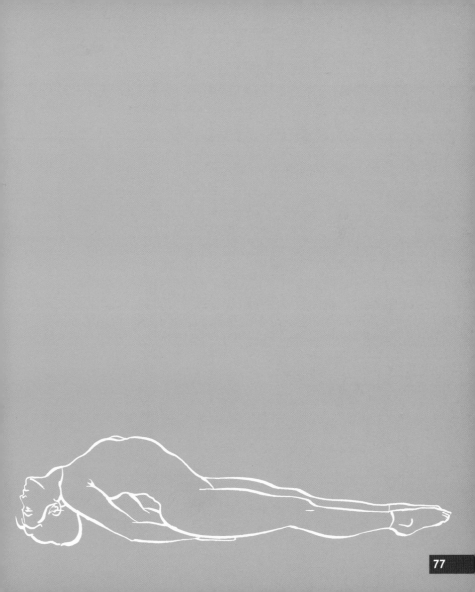

❶ Focus your breath

Improves circulation to all organs • Relaxes muscles and ligaments •
Relieves stress

Lie down and gently close your eyes. Slowly inhale through the nose and focus on your breath as it travels down the throat and into the bottom of the lungs and ribcage. Be aware of your lungs and ribcage expanding and your spine lengthening. You will feel the abdomen rise.

Exhale through your nose. Feel the abdomen fall. The out-breath should be longer than the in-breath.

Surrender the weight of your body into the ground. Let go of your thoughts. Focus your breathing.

- The exhalation holds the key to relaxation. The more stale air you exhale, the more fresh air you can inhale, the deeper your breathing, the quieter the mind.

  Focus your breath ... relax ... relax.

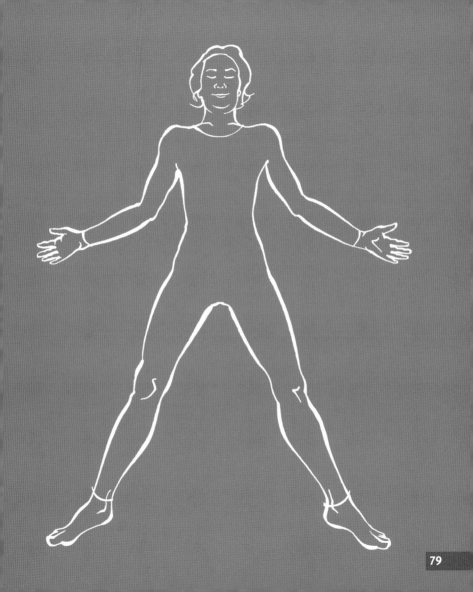

❷ The cobbler

Improves circulation to all organs • Stretches the inner thighs and groin • Opens the chest and shoulders • Helps to relieve asthma and menstrual discomfort

1 Lie on your back and bend your knees up towards the ceiling so that your feet are a few inches away from your buttocks, your feet and ankles together. Spread your arms to an angle of 45 degrees to your body. Keep your head centred and your chin tucked in. Inhale to prepare.

2 As you slowly exhale, begin to open your knees.

3 Continue to open your knees, keeping the lower back pressed into the ground.

▶ Focus your breath as you allow the hips to open fully. Hold for 1 minute. Then slowly bring the knees together.

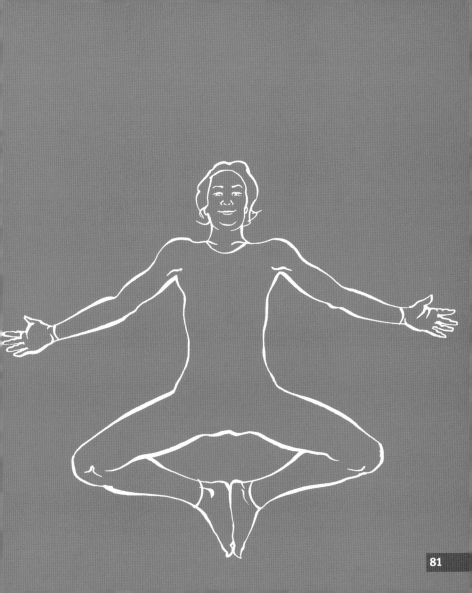

❸ The hip roll

Stimulates the liver, kidneys and intestines • Helps to relieve trapped nerves, indigestion and constipation • Stretches the thighs • Releases tension in the spine • Opens the shoulders and chest • Helps to relieve asthma

Caution: Do not attempt this posture if you are pregnant.

1 Lying on your back, feet together, bend your knees up to the ceiling. Bring your arms out, level with your shoulders, palms facing up. Your head should be centred and your chin tucked in. Inhale to prepare.

2 As you slowly exhale, drop your knees to the left as far as is comfortable. As you do so, turn your head to the right, twisting the spine.

3 Inhale. Then slowly exhale, bringing the knees and head back to centre.

▶ Repeat to the other side. Continue for 2 minutes, twisting to one side then the other. To finish, bring the knees and head back to centre.

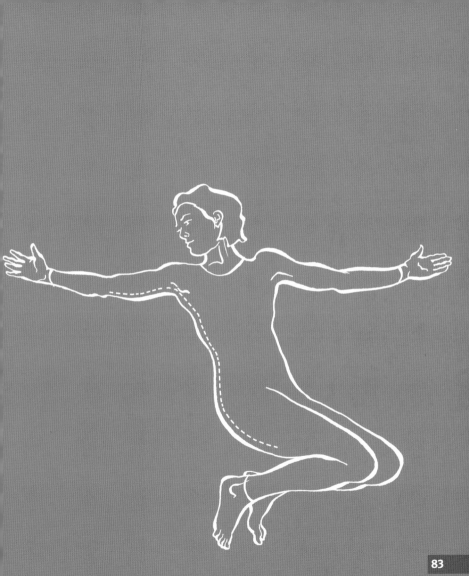

83

④ The pelvic tilt

Stimulates the thyroid • Expands the lungs • Stretches the neck and thighs • Strengthens the lower back and abdominal muscles • Helps to relieve asthma, menstrual discomfort and back pain

Caution: Avoid this posture if you're pregnant or have a neck injury.

1 Lie on your back with your knees bent and your feet hip-width apart, heels turned out slightly. Place your arms by your sides, palms down. Keep your head centred and your chin tucked in. Inhale to prepare.

2 Slowly exhale, lifting your tail bone off the ground as you do so.

3 Lift each vertebra off the ground one by one until you reach the shoulder blades.

▶ Root your feet firmly into the ground. Become aware of your chest opening as you push the spine up as far as is comfortable. Inhale. Then exhale as you slowly lower the spine, one vertebra at a time – upper spine, central spine, lower spine, tail bone. Repeat the pelvic tilt for 1 minute.

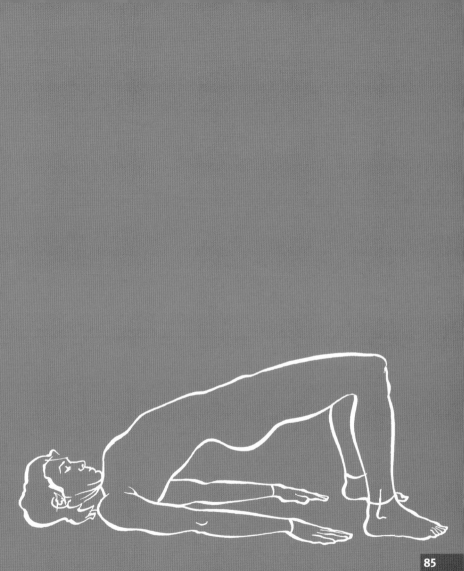

❺ The big toe

Improves circulation to all organs • Stretches the hamstrings and calf muscles • Tones the abdominal muscles • Improves flexibility in the hips • Helps to relieve back pain, indigestion and constipation

1 Lie on your back with your chin tucked into your neck, and your lower back pressed into the ground. Inhale to prepare.

2 Slowly exhale, raising your legs off the ground. Use your hands to support your upper legs.

3 Focusing your breath, raise the legs as far as you can manage, using your hands to guide them. Extend through the heels to open up the backs of the legs.

▶ Grab hold of your toes and gently pull your legs towards you as far as is comfortable, keeping the backs of the knees open. Hold the posture for 1 minute. Slowly lower your legs to the floor.

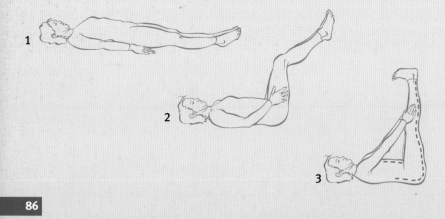

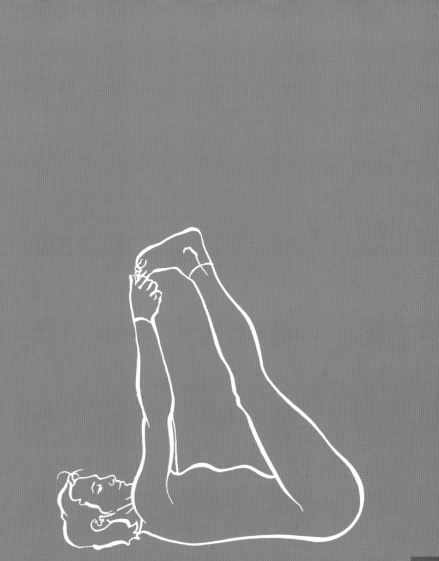

⑥ The half dog

Stimulates the liver, kidneys and intestines • Helps to relieve lower back pain and indigestion • Tones the arms • Opens the chest, central spine and shoulders • Helps to relieve asthma

1 On all fours, position your hands in line with the shoulders, and your knees hip-width apart. Inhale to prepare.

2 As you exhale, widen the arms and move them forwards on the floor.

3 Slowly drop the chest and shoulders towards the ground, ensuring that the hips remain in line with the knees.

▶ Focus your breath, allowing the chest and shoulders to open and the spine to lengthen. Hold the posture for 1 minute, or less if it becomes uncomfortable. Then return to the starting position.

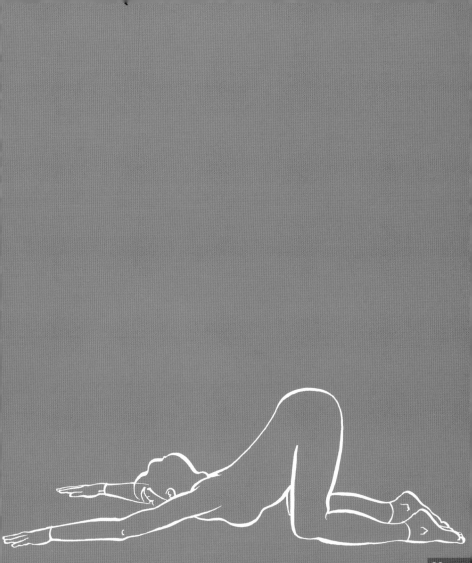

❼ The cobra

Improves circulation to all organs • Tones the arms and abdomen •
Expands the lungs • Helps to relieve asthma, menstrual discomfort,
constipation and indigestion

Caution: Avoid this posture if you're pregnant or suffer from lower back pain.

1 Lie on your front with your forehead down, legs together and hands
   in line with the outside of your shoulders. Inhale to prepare.

2 As you exhale, slowly lift the forehead, chin and neck, pushing your
   hands into the ground.

3 Continue to push, lifting the chest and ribs. Draw the elbows down
   towards the waist, pull the shoulders back and down, and open the chest.

▶ Focus your breath. Hold the posture for 30 seconds. Then slowly lower
   the ribs, chest, neck, chin and finally the forehead, back to the floor.
   Then repeat.

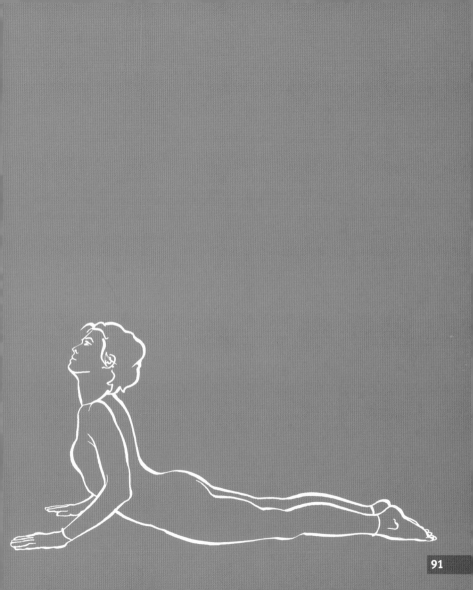

❽ The mountain

Improves circulation to all organs • Tones the arms • Firms the abdomen • Improves posture

1 Stand with your feet hip-width apart, heels turned out slightly. Stretch your arms out in front of you and link your fingers.

2 Inhale to prepare.

3 As you exhale, stretch your arms up above your head and root your feet firmly into the ground. Become aware of the opposite stretch creating space around your waist.

▶ Focus your breath as you stretch gently in the posture. Hold the stretch for 1 minute. Then release your arms and place them by your sides.

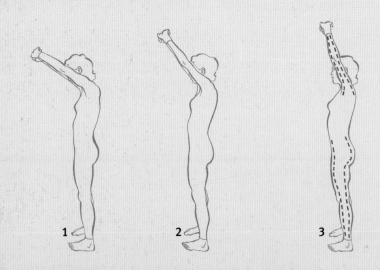

1   2   3

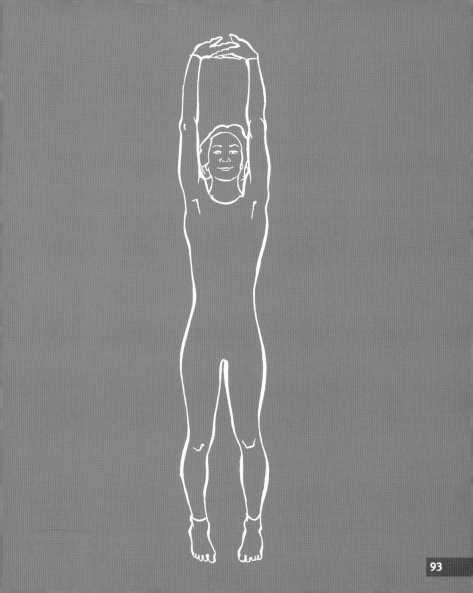

❾ The stork

Improves circulation to all organs • Stretches the thighs and arms •
Expands the lungs • Opens the hips • Helps to relieve asthma and stress
• Improves concentration and balance

1   Stand with your feet hip-width apart, toes pointing forwards, arms by
    your sides.

2   Bend your right leg up behind you and take hold of the ankle with your
    right hand. Raise your left arm so that your fingers point towards the
    ceiling. Your arm should gently brush your ear. Inhale to prepare.

3   Root the left foot firmly into the ground and, as you exhale, slowly lean
    forwards and push your right foot up to the ceiling. Make sure your
    hips are straight throughout – do not allow them to twist. Keep the
    grounded leg strong and straight.

▶   Focus your breath. Hold the posture for 1 minute. Then slowly release
    the leg, and relax the arm. Repeat to the other side.

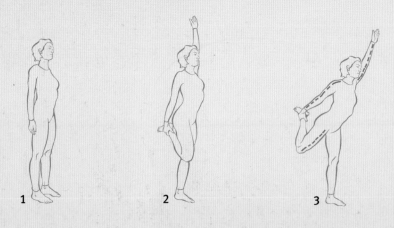

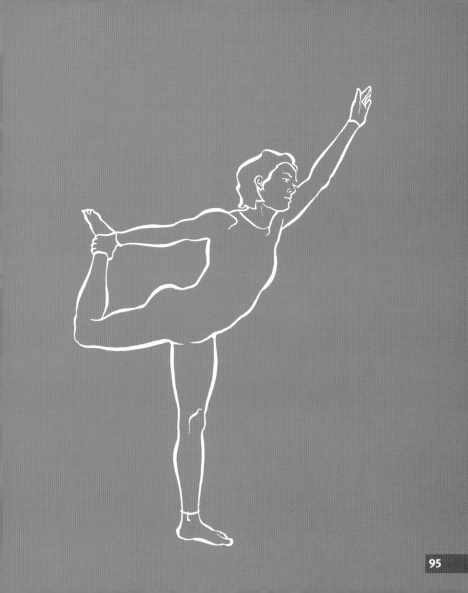

⑩ The shoulder stand

Improves circulation to all organs • Stretches the neck • Stimulates the thyroid • Invigorates the body • Tones the abdominal muscles • Helps to relieve asthma, indigestion and varicose veins

Caution: Avoid this posture if you're pregnant or suffering from high blood pressure, neck pain or injury, or pins and needles in the arms or hands.

1   Lie on your back with your legs together, arms by your sides, palms face down. Keep your head centred and your chin tucked in. Inhale to prepare.

2   As you exhale, slowly raise your legs until they're positioned over your torso. Then, pressing your hands into the floor, begin to lift your hips.

3   Support your back with both hands, fingers turned into the spine, thumbs around the hips. Continue to lift the legs and hips, gradually moving the hands up the back as the distance between your head and feet increases. Keep your elbows tucked in to distribute the weight evenly and avoid pressure on the neck and shoulders.

▶   Focus your breath. Hold the posture for 1–2 minutes, or less if it becomes uncomfortable. To release, slowly take your legs to an angle of 45 degrees over your head, and press your palms into the floor. Slowly lower the spine to the floor, one vertebra at a time, followed by the legs.

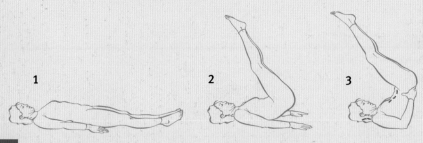

1   2   3

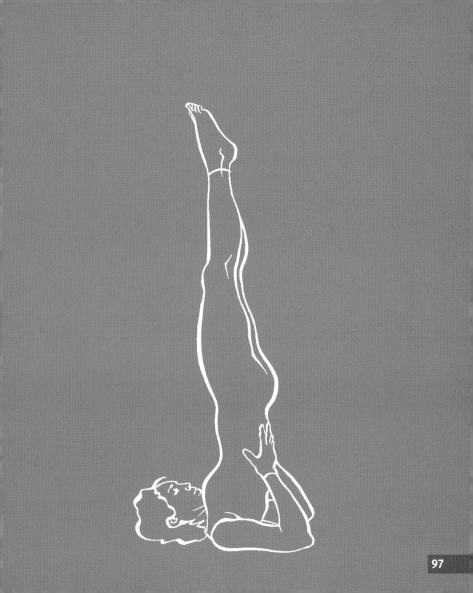

⑪ The plough

Improves circulation to all organs • Stretches the neck, spine, hamstrings and calf muscles • Stimulates the thyroid • Helps to relieve asthma, neck and back pain, indigestion and constipation

Caution: Avoid this posture if you're pregnant or suffering from high blood pressure, neck pain or injury, or pins and needles in the arms or hands.

1 Lie on your back with your legs together. Place your arms by your sides, palms down. Your head should be centred, chin tucked in. Inhale.

2 As you exhale, press your hands into the ground. Slowly raise your legs until they're positioned over your torso, then raise your hips.

3 Support your back with both hands, fingers turned into the spine and thumbs towards the hips. Tuck your elbows in. Slowly take your legs over your head. The aim is for your feet to touch the floor behind your head, but do not force them if it starts to feel uncomfortable.

▶ Tuck your toes in and straighten your legs. Keep the hips lifted and the chin tucked in to take the weight away from the neck and shoulders. Focus your breath. Hold the posture for 1 minute. To release, press your palms into the floor, then slowly lower the spine one vertebra at a time from the shoulders to the tail bone. Then gently lower the legs.

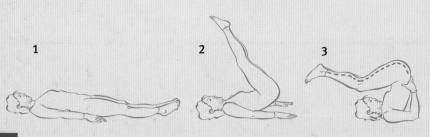

1

2

3

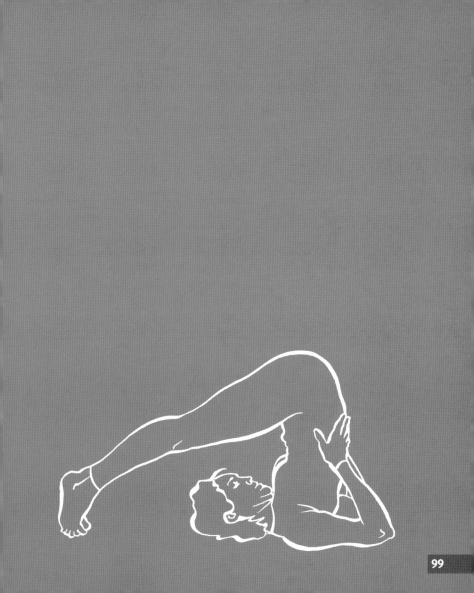

⑫ The fish

Expands the lungs • Stimulates the thyroid • Stretches the neck and spine •
Opens the shoulders • Tones the arms • Helps to relieve asthma and stress

Caution: Avoid this posture if you have a neck injury or suffer from pins and needles in the arms or hands.

1 Lie on your back with your legs together. Place your arms by your sides, palms down. Keep your head centred, chin tucked in.

2 With your arms straight, position your hands underneath your buttocks so that your hands are side by side, pointing towards the thighs. Inhale to prepare.

3 Exhale, pressing your elbows into the floor. As you do so, arch your back and lift your chest.

▶ Slowly lower your head back until the top of the head touches the floor. Focus your breath. Hold the posture for 1 minute. To release, gently lift your head, then lower your body, returning your arms to your sides.

1

2

3

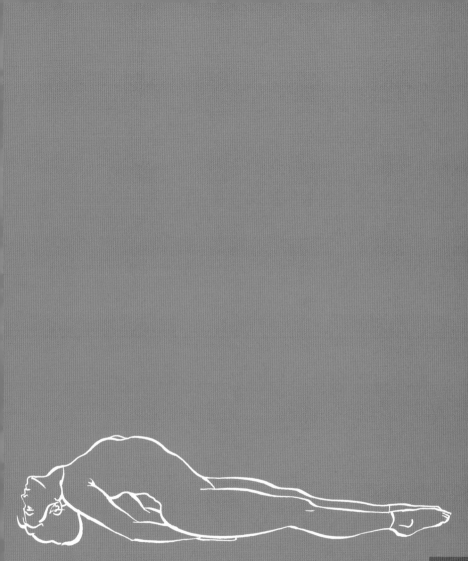

wake up
and let go

10-MINUTE SESSIONS

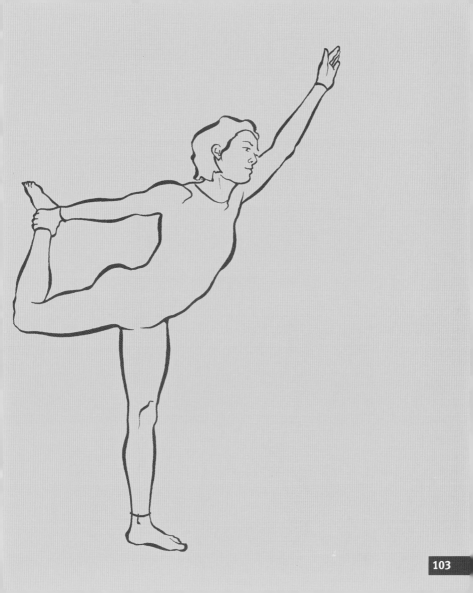

❶ The mountain

Improves circulation to all organs • Tones the arms • Firms the abdomen • Improves posture

1 Stand with your feet hip-width apart, heels turned out slightly. Stretch your arms out in front of you and link your fingers.

2 Inhale to prepare.

3 As you exhale, stretch your arms up above your head and root your feet firmly into the ground. Become aware of the opposite stretch creating space around your waist.

▶ Focus your breath as you stretch gently in the posture. Hold the stretch for 1 minute. Then release your arms and place them by your sides.

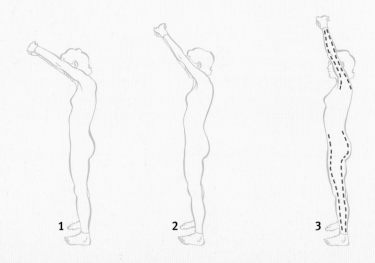

1   2   3

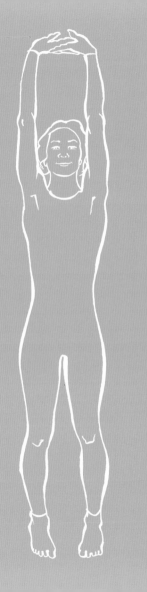

② Letting go

Stimulates the liver, kidneys and intestines • Helps to relieve stress, fatigue and indigestion • Stretches the calf muscles and hamstrings

Caution: Do not attempt this posture if you suffer from high blood pressure.

1 Standing with your feet hip-width apart and your heels turned out slightly, relax your body forwards, your arms hanging down.

2 Inhale as your body relaxes down.

3 As you exhale, drop your chin to your chest and slowly continue to release your spine, one vertebra at a time. Do not bounce. Root your feet firmly into the ground to keep your legs strong, and open the backs of the knees without locking them. Let go of the tension in the upper body.

▶ Exhale to release the spine, then the shoulders, arms, fingers, neck, face, jaw and eyes. Focus your breath as you hold the posture. Hold for 1 minute, then slowly come up to a standing position.

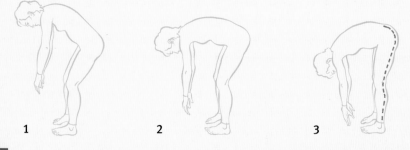

1   2   3

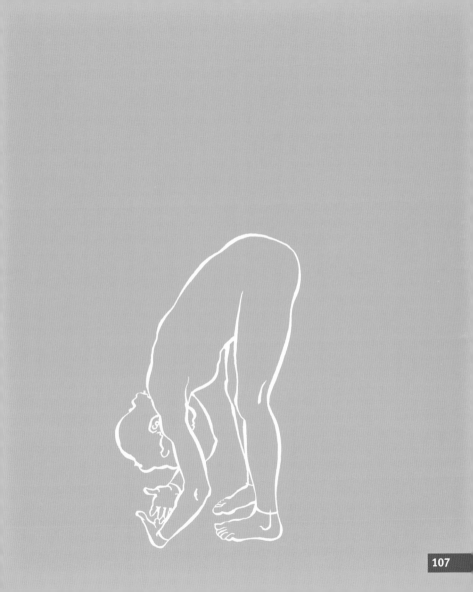

❸ The standing fish

Corrects rounded shoulders • Expands lungs • Tones the arms • Helps to relieve asthma, lethargy and anxiety

1 Standing with your feet hip-width apart, heels turned out slightly, link your fingers together behind your back.

2 Inhale to prepare.

3 As you exhale, slowly lift the centre of the chest and open the shoulders back, pulling the arms down. Root your feet firmly into the ground, keeping your legs strong and the backs of the knees open.

▶ As you focus your breath in the posture, your chest should be lifted and fully open and your arms pulled back. Hold for 1 minute. Then slowly release your arms and allow them to rest by your sides.

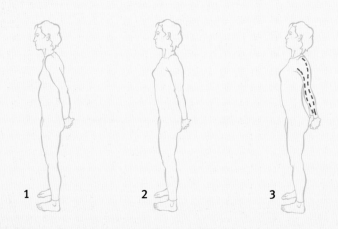

1   2   3

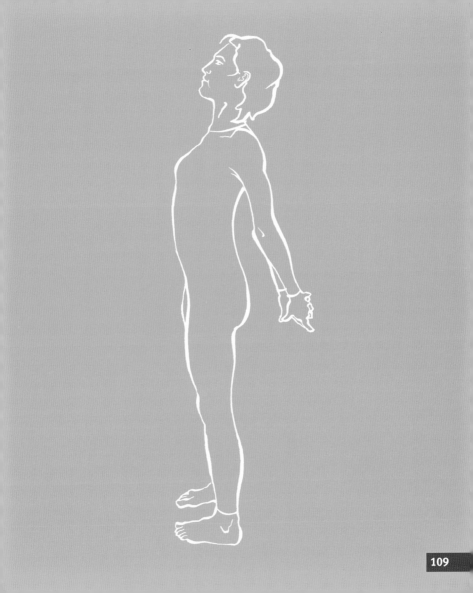

❹ The triangle variation

Stimulates the kidneys, liver and intestines • Helps to relieve fatigue, stress, stiffness in the shoulders and indigestion • Stretches the calf muscles and hamstrings • Tones the arms

Caution: Do not attempt this posture if you suffer from high blood pressure or lower back pain.

1 Stand with your feet wide apart, toes pointing forwards. Root your feet firmly into the ground. Position your hands behind your back and link your fingers together. Inhale to prepare.

2 As you exhale, slowly bend forwards with the spine relaxed.

3 Continue to bend, taking your arms over your head.

▶ Focus your breath. Hold the posture for 1 minute. Then slowly return to the standing position and release the arms.

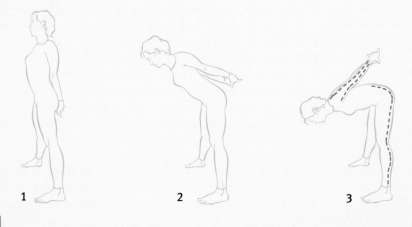

1   2   3

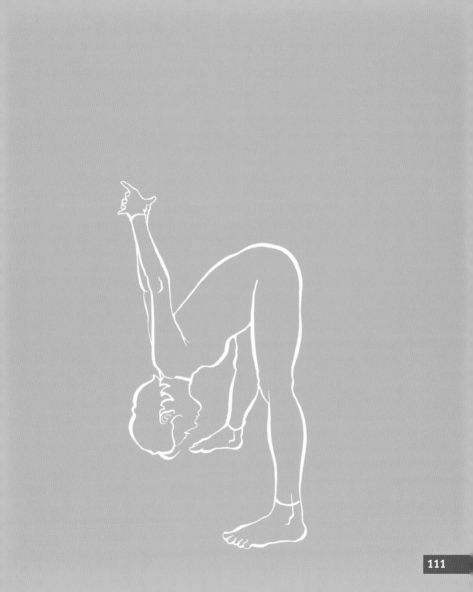

⑤ The wide-leg triangle

Stimulates the liver, kidneys and intestines • Helps to relieve indigestion • Improves balance and spinal flexibility • Tones the legs • Stretches the arms • Strengthens the lower back and abdominal muscles

1 Stand with your feet wide apart, toes pointing forwards. Raise your right arm so that it brushes against your ear, fingers pointing to the ceiling. Inhale to prepare.

2 With your face turned into the raised arm, slowly exhale. As you do so, stretch your arm and torso to the left, keeping the left arm straight, by your side.

3 As you stretch, root your right foot firmly into the ground. Ensure that your hips are pointing forwards – do not allow them to twist. If you experience any pain in your sides, stop.

▶ Focus your breath. Hold the posture for 30 seconds. Then slowly return to the standing position and release the arm. Repeat to the other side.

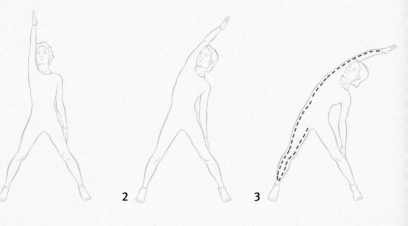

1   2   3

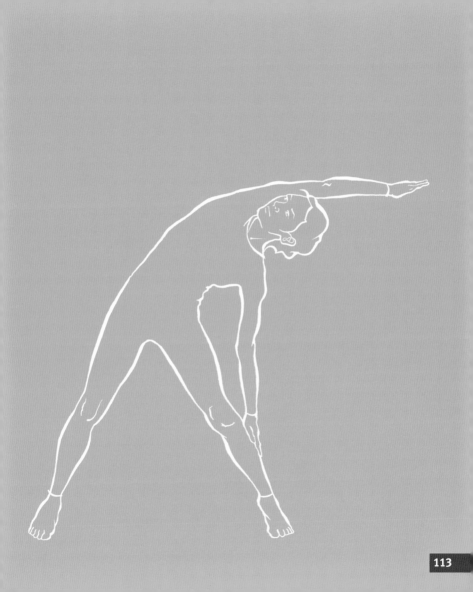

⑥ The dog

Improves circulation to all organs • Stretches the calf muscles, hamstrings, spine, arms and hands • Helps to relieve back pain, headache, fatigue and indigestion

Caution: Do not attempt this posture if you have high blood pressure.

1   On all fours, position your hands in line with the shoulders, knees hip-width apart. Inhale to prepare.

2   As you exhale, bring your weight onto the toes, and slowly lift the knees.

3   Push your tail bone up and out. With your heels turned outwards slightly, extend them to the floor to open out the backs of the knees.

▶   Lengthening the legs fully, relax the neck and face. Focus your breath. Hold the posture for 1 minute. Then slowly return to the starting position.

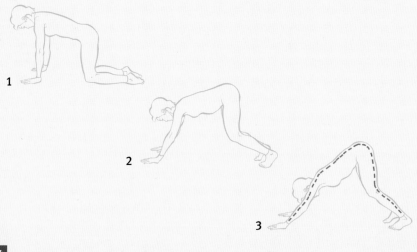

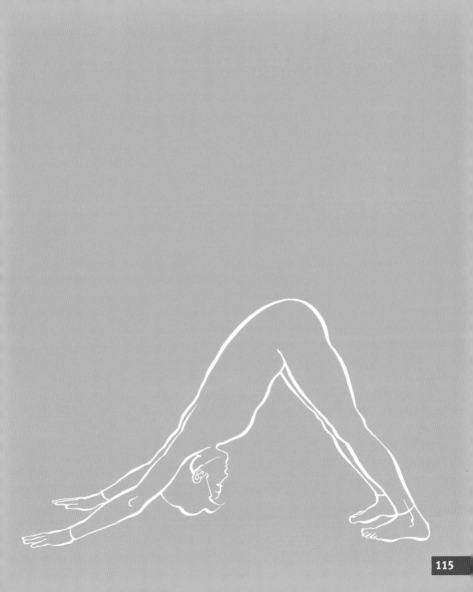

❶ Focus your breath

Improves circulation to all organs • Relaxes muscles and ligaments • Relieves stress

Lie down and gently close your eyes. Slowly inhale through the nose and focus on your breath as it travels down the throat and into the bottom of the lungs and ribcage. Be aware of your lungs and ribcage expanding and your spine lengthening. You will feel the abdomen rise.

Exhale through your nose. Feel the abdomen fall. The out-breath should be longer than the in-breath.

Surrender the weight of your body into the ground. Let go of your thoughts. Focus your breathing.

- **The exhalation holds the key to relaxation. The more stale air you exhale, the more fresh air you can inhale, the deeper your breathing, the quieter the mind.**

  Focus your breath ... relax ... relax.

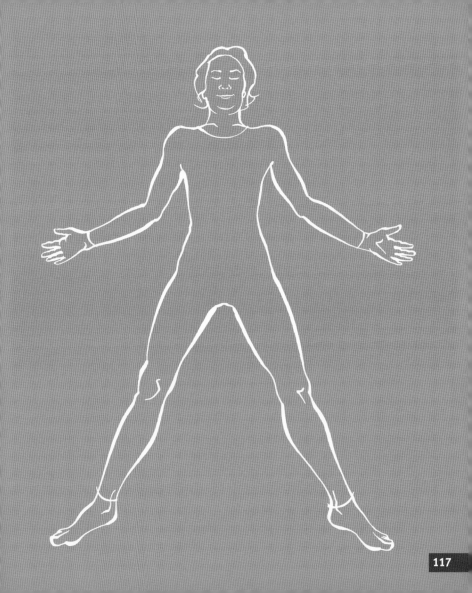

② The cobbler

Improves circulation to all organs • Stretches the inner thighs and groin •
Opens the chest and shoulders • Helps to relieve asthma and menstrual
discomfort

1 Lie on your back and bend your knees up towards the ceiling so that
   your feet are a few inches away from your buttocks, your feet and ankles
   together. Spread your arms to an angle of 45 degrees to your body. Keep
   your head centred and your chin tucked in. Inhale to prepare.

2 As you slowly exhale, begin to open your knees.

3 Continue to open your knees, keeping the lower back pressed into the
   ground.

▶ Focus your breath as you allow the hips to open fully. Hold for
   1 minute. Then slowly bring the knees together.

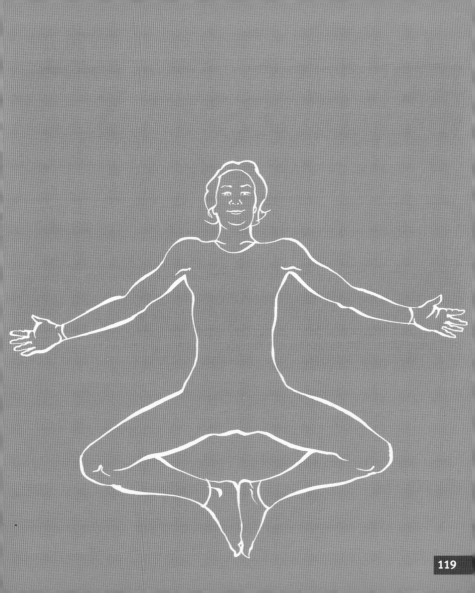

❸ The hip roll

Stimulates the liver, kidneys and intestines • Helps to relieve trapped nerves, indigestion and constipation • Stretches the thighs • Releases tension in the spine • Opens the shoulders and chest • Helps to relieve asthma

Caution: Do not attempt this posture if you are pregnant.

1 Lying on your back, feet together, bend your knees up to the ceiling. Bring your arms out, level with your shoulders, palms facing up. Your head should be centred and your chin tucked in. Inhale to prepare.

2 As you slowly exhale, drop your knees to the left as far as is comfortable. As you do so, turn your head to the right, twisting the spine.

3 Inhale. Then slowly exhale, bringing the knees and head back to centre.

▶ Repeat to the other side. Continue for 2 minutes, twisting to one side then the other. To finish, bring the knees and head back to centre.

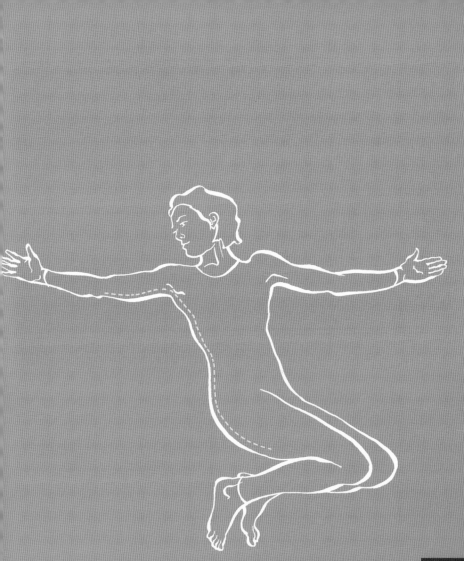

❹ The pelvic tilt

Stimulates the thyroid • Expands the lungs • Stretches the neck and thighs • Strengthens the lower back and abdominal muscles • Helps to relieve asthma, menstrual discomfort and back pain

Caution: Avoid this posture if you're pregnant or have a neck injury.

1 Lie on your back with your knees bent and your feet hip-width apart, heels turned out slightly. Place your arms by your sides, palms down. Keep your head centred and your chin tucked in. Inhale to prepare.

2 Slowly exhale, lifting your tail bone off the ground as you do so.

3 Lift each vertebra off the ground one by one until you reach the shoulder blades.

▶ Root your feet firmly into the ground. Become aware of your chest opening as you push the spine up as far as is comfortable. Inhale. Then exhale as you slowly lower the spine, one vertebra at a time – upper spine, central spine, lower spine, tail bone. Repeat the pelvic tilt for 1 minute.

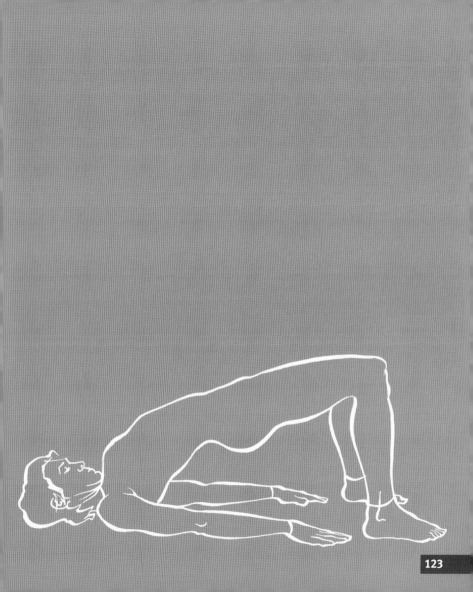

❺ The big toe

Improves circulation to all organs • Stretches the hamstrings and calf muscles • Tones the abdominal muscles • Improves flexibility in the hips • Helps to relieve back pain, indigestion and constipation

1 Lie on your back with your chin tucked into your neck, and your lower back pressed into the ground. Inhale to prepare.

2 Slowly exhale, raising your legs off the ground. Use your hands to support your upper legs.

3 Focusing your breath, raise the legs as far as you can manage, using your hands to guide them. Extend through the heels to open up the backs of the legs.

▶ Grab hold of your toes and gently pull your legs towards you as far as is comfortable, keeping the backs of the knees open. Hold the posture for 1 minute. Slowly lower your legs to the floor.

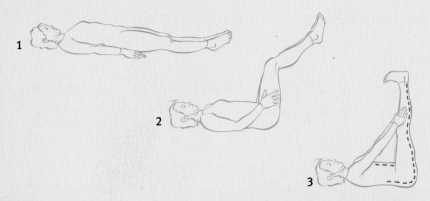

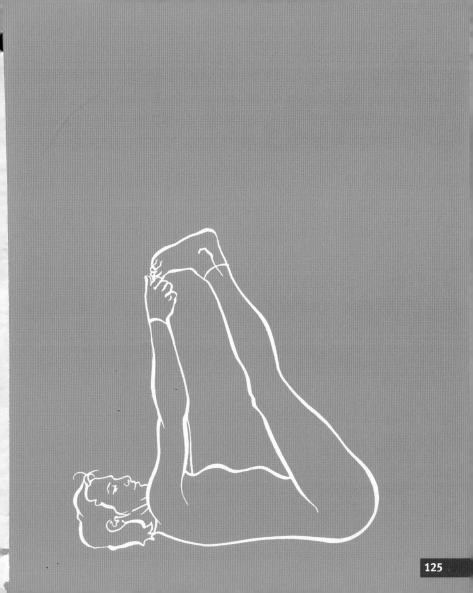

❻ The stork

*Improves circulation to all organs • Stretches the thighs and arms •
Expands the lungs • Opens the hips • Helps to relieve asthma and stress
• Improves concentration and balance*

1 Stand with your feet hip-width apart, toes pointing forwards, arms by
   your sides.

2 Bend your right leg up behind you and take hold of the ankle with your
   right hand. Raise your left arm so that your fingers point towards the
   ceiling. Your arm should gently brush your ear. Inhale to prepare.

3 Root the left foot firmly into the ground and, as you exhale, slowly lean
   forwards and push your right foot up to the ceiling. Make sure your
   hips are straight throughout – do not allow them to twist. Keep the
   grounded leg strong and straight.

▶ Focus your breath. Hold the posture for 1 minute. Then slowly release
   the leg, and relax the arm. Repeat to the other side.

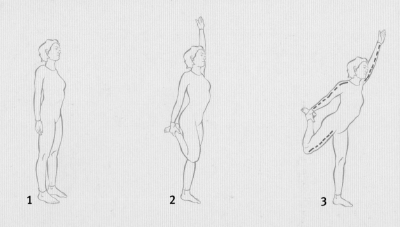

1   2   3

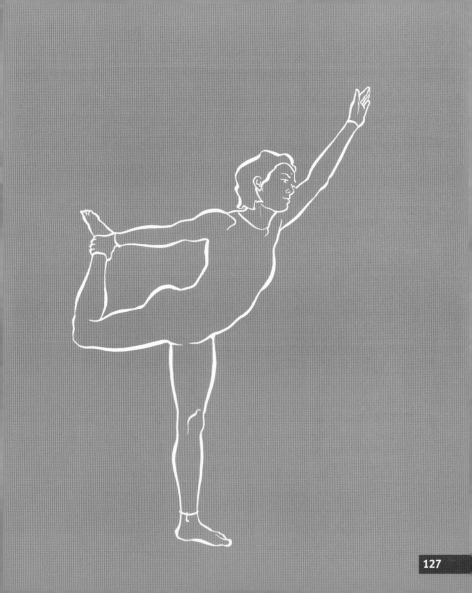

ABOUT THE AUTHOR

Jude Reignier is an experienced yoga teacher living and working in Notting Hill, London. She trained at the Shivananda Yoga Centre in the Catskills, New York, where she was awarded an excellent diploma. During the last ten years of teaching she has developed her own individual style based on the knowledge she has gained working with people on a one-to-one basis, with various groups, with children and those with special needs. Jude is married and has two children.

ABOUT THE CONSULTANT

Sean Durkan has a BSc degree from the London School of Osteopathy, and is a member of the General Osteopathic Council. He has been in practice for seven years at Harley Street, London, and he also has residency at the Queen's Tennis Club, London, where he treats sports professionals; his clients also include many actors and musicians. Sean takes a holistic approach to osteopathy, looking at clients' posture, dietary habits and general lifestyle as a way to improve well-being. His personal interests include yoga and pilates.

ACKNOWLEDGEMENTS

Very special thanks to my husband Tristan, without whose love and artistic skills I couldn't have done this book. To my son Natty and daughter Dionne for their patience. Thanks to Simon Trewin for recommending Robert Smith Literary Agency and Robert for his continual support. I am very grateful to Eddison Sadd for publishing my book, and especially to Ian Jackson, Elaine Partington, Katie Golsby and Malcolm Smythe for all their hard work. Thanks to Sean Durkan for his advice and support on the introduction and internal organs. To Juliet Percival for the great illustrations, all my clients for their encouragement and inspiration, especially Bertie Newbery (Milk Studios), Ingrid Western, Jackie Hyde and Elaine Maley (Natural Healing Centre). Finally, thank you to my dad, mum and sisters.